T0234717

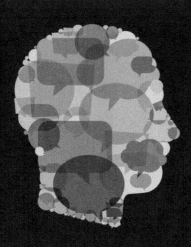

DIAGNOSTIC
REPORT WRITING
IN SPEECH-LANGUAGE PATHOLOGY
A Guide to Effective Communication

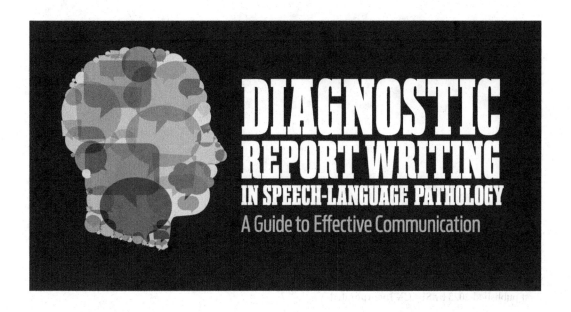

DIAGNOSTIC REPORT WRITING
IN SPEECH-LANGUAGE PATHOLOGY
A Guide to Effective Communication

STEVEN H. BLAUSTEIN, PhD, CCC-SLP, BCS-CL
ASSOCIATE PROFESSOR
GRADUATE PROGRAM IN SPEECH-LANGUAGE PATHOLOGY
SCHOOL OF HEALTH SCIENCES
TOURO UNIVERSITY
NEW YORK, NEW YORK

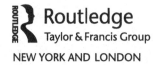

Routledge
Taylor & Francis Group

NEW YORK AND LONDON

First published 2023 by SLACK Incorporated

Published in 2024 by Routledge
605 Third Avenue, New York, NY 10158

and by Routledge
4 Park Square, Milton Park, Abingdon, Oxon, OX14 4RN

Routledge is an imprint of the Taylor & Francis Group, an informa business

© 2023 by Taylor & Francis Group

Dr. Steven H. Blaustein reported no financial or proprietary interest in the materials presented herein. *Gary S. Mayerson* has not reported any financial or proprietary interest in the materials presented herein.

Cover Artist: Tinhouse Design

Library of Congress Control Number: 2022945303

ISBN: 9781630918873 (pbk)
ISBN: 9781003523833 (ebk)

DOI: 10.4324/9781003523833

Dedication

This book is dedicated to my son, Eric Jon Blaustein. He was kind, generous, funny, intelligent, and wise. He was truly my friend. Eric was a dedicated and loving son, husband, father, brother, and friend. His strength and courage were an inspiration to all who had the privilege of knowing him. There are no words to describe how he will be forever missed. His time with us was way too short.

To my wife, Ellen, and my son, Robert, both of whom I love and respect to no end. They are constantly giving of themselves and helping to make the world whole.

With deep gratitude.

Contents

ABOUT THE AUTHOR

Steven H. Blaustein, PhD, CCC-SLP, BCS-CL, holds a Certificate of Clinical Competence in Speech-Language Pathology from the American Speech-Language-Hearing Association (ASHA) and is a Board-Certified Specialist in Child Language with more than 50 years of clinical experience. He holds a doctorate degree in Speech and Hearing Sciences from the Graduate Center of the City University of New York.

Dr. Blaustein's experience includes 18 years at Mount Sinai Hospital in New York where, in addition to providing clinical services for children and adult inpatients and outpatients, Dr. Blaustein spent 4 years as the coordinator and consulting speech-language pathologist to the Cleft Palate and Craniofacial Disorders Center. He directed a hospital-based program for speech and language disorders and has consulted for a variety of programs and agencies. This work included completing thousands of evaluations for the New York State Early Intervention Program and numerous preschool programs serving New York City Committees on Preschool Special Education. He continues to advocate for individuals with communication disorders and routinely conducts independent speech and language evaluations and presents his findings and opinions at impartial hearings and has testified in court. Dr. Blaustein has presented numerous continuing education workshops, seminars, and lectures on various speech- and language-related topics throughout the United States, including frequent presentations at annual conventions of the ASHA. Dr. Blaustein has served on advisory boards for social skills programs and therapeutic schools for children with communication disorders. He has had papers published in *Neurology* and *Journal of Communication Disorders* and contributed a chapter to *ALS: A Guide to Patient Care*. Dr. Blaustein reviews assessment instruments and textbooks related to language disorders for various publishers. His current interests are in the areas of evaluation and diagnosis of communication disorders, autism, social pragmatic language disorders, speech sound production, Early Intervention, and interprofessional education.

Dr. Blaustein has served as Adjunct Clinical Professor at a number of colleges and universities and is currently a full-time Associate Professor at the Touro University School of Health Sciences Graduate Program in Speech-Language Pathology. He continues to maintain a private practice specializing in the assessment of toddlers and children.

FOREWORD

In the world of the licensed and certified speech-language pathologist, diagnostics is where the rehabilitation process begins. The preparation of the diagnostic report, however, is a process that, at least historically, has allowed tremendous variations in style, form, and content. For better or for worse, well-intentioned speech-language pathologists writing diagnostic reports are, on each occasion, reinventing the wheel.

At first blush, the active practitioner might be tempted to embrace having so much latitude and flexibility. Dr. Blaustein, however, makes the compelling case that employing high and consistent standards and ensuring accountability is absolutely essential where, as is often the case, the patient is seeking funding for services or a therapeutic placement, or is pursuing some other objective requiring an authorization, court order, or other stamp of approval.

As Dr. Blaustein goes on to explain, writing a diagnostic report is not just about measuring and presenting test scores. The end product of diagnostics must be a thorough, professional, and ethical evaluation report where the clinician has viewed the process through a wide lens that has included the perspective of the patient and the family. Ultimately, subject to any restrictions or limitations imposed by an employer, the evaluator is left with the final decision as to what to include, what to leave out, what recommendations to make, and generally how to make sense of it all for the betterment of the patient.

The diagnostic report can contain technical jargon, so long as that jargon is presented so as to be understandable by a reader who is not working in the field. The best diagnostic reports are those that cut through the many moving pieces to point the patient's services in the right direction.

It can be a serious mistake to regard the diagnostic report as something that will be read and then filed away in a dusty file cabinet, never to be seen again. As Dr. Blaustein explains, it should be anticipated that today's diagnostic report may surface to become the focus of attention in a variety of judicial and administrative proceedings. Your professional reputation can turn on not only what you say, but how you say it. Moreover, while this might seem manifestly unfair, your diagnostic report may be reviewed years after the fact with the benefit of 20/20 hindsight.

Every recommendation in a report matters. Indeed, every word in a report matters. Having worked with Dr. Blaustein for more than 20 years, and having qualified him as an expert in a variety of court settings, I can attest to the fact that his evidence-based diagnostic reports and professional recommendations have been able to withstand the test of time.

Dr. Blaustein has written what undoubtedly will be considered the definitive guide to preparing and writing diagnostic reports. More important, Dr. Blaustein's guide raises the bar in a big way for patients and family members who are seeking individualized and effective interventions.

—*Gary S. Mayerson, JD*

Gary S. Mayerson, JD, is the founder of Mayerson & Associates, the first law firm in the nation dedicated to the representation of individuals diagnosed on the autism spectrum. He is responsible for more than 150 federal court decisions, including the first autism case to reach the U.S. Supreme Court. He is the author of *Autism's Declaration of Independence* and *How to Compromise With Your School District Without Compromising Your Child*.

Introduction

During the more than 50 years that I have worked as a clinician, evaluator, college professor, consultant, administrator, and clinical supervisor, the one aspect of our profession that most often brings frowns to the faces of most students and colleagues is the topic of clinical diagnostic report writing. For students, it may be the amount of time necessary to learn the report writing process and the hours spent writing and rewriting reports editing, critiquing, and perhaps even grading by faculty and supervisors. The sheer enormity of the tasks can be overwhelming. For others, it can be learning to administer the various "tests," scoring them, interpreting results, and considering recommendations.

Admittedly, too little time is spent in graduate programs on the important skill of diagnostic report writing, and most graduate students in speech-language pathology programs are lucky if they get to complete even a handful of written diagnostic evaluations during their entire academic career. It is not enough. Yet, the knowledge and skills involved in clinical writing and documentation are as important as any other area learned. They are actually becoming more important in the current era of ever-increasing accountability, oversight, and regulation.

For speech-language pathology graduates beginning their careers and entering Clinical Fellowship programs, time is further spent learning and refining diagnostic skills and learning these tasks under the tutelage and supervision of a more experienced mentor. They are still required to maintain a caseload, provide therapy, attend important meetings, complete necessary paperwork, and do this under the umbrella of a new work setting where greater independence and demands are required. Again, the time spent learning to complete evaluations can be limited and the additional time spent completing the edits, rewrites, and changes asked for by supervisors can be challenging. Even the experienced clinician will often state, "I just don't like testing and the writing, it's not my thing." Perhaps it is having to keep up with new assessment instruments that are constantly being published and have to be studied, practiced, and learned that can be overwhelming. Maybe it is keeping abreast of the frequent revisions of already existing tests that we have become all too famil-iar with. It may be the time involved in having administration, scoring, test interpretation, analysis, conclusions, and eventually putting this all to paper. This is often under a time constraint as our patients, clients, various school and clinic supervisors, and third-party payers are always asking, "Is the report ready yet?" It is no wonder that while most clinicians will readily and cheerfully proclaim how they love therapy, their patients and clients, and working with language, fluency, aphasia, or phonology, the clinicians that tell you they love diagnostics and the subsequent report writing can be few and far between.

The author of this book is one such clinician who enjoys clinical diagnostic evaluation report writing. I hope to show in the pages that follow that the assessment of a communication disorder, fully understanding its nature, and providing that insight to a patient or client, their families, and allied professionals can be one of the most rewarding, stimulating, and professionally satisfying as-pects of our career. It calls into play all of our knowledge, experience, and insight, and the result, if successfully accomplished, can be life altering for the individuals we work with that seek our help. The diagnosis is where the rehabilitation process begins. We see our patients at the most difficult times and hopefully begin to answer some questions, provide some support, and shed some light on the future and, whether promising or uncertain, provide a prognosis that will enable our patients to face the future understanding their communication difficulty and the impact it will have on their lives. The diagnostic evaluation report is the culmination of the evaluation process. The report is an important legal document that has multiple functions, that by law must be made available for years, and serves as the basis for the initiation of processes from intervention planning to reimbursement for services.

This book will present the diagnostic report as the end product of a logical process. As in every other aspect of our profession, it requires a specific set of knowledge and skills. A process that, if understood and correctly used, will hopefully make the evaluation and subsequent writing and presentation of a professional written document more meaningful, less cumbersome, and even more exciting. At the very least, I hope to make the writing process clearer. An evaluation consists of numerous parts. It is a sequence of steps that must be followed with each step leading to the next. When properly placed together and documented, the ensuing report is a reflection and testimony to these steps. This book will take you through each step of the process, chapter by chapter, in the order in which a speech and language evaluation is conducted. It reflects our skill, training, ability, and where we are professionally. We should be adept at completing a professional diagnostic evaluation and proud to present a finished document that is not only beneficial to our patients and clients but also makes us stand out as accomplished professionals. It is important to remember that the end of every report bears our name and signature. It is the last thing a reader will see and the first thing they will remember if a report is well written and useful or contains errors or is insufficient and results in problems.

The information presented in this book is based on having completed thousands of diagnostic evaluations of communication disorders over years of practice. It will bring together the science and art of assessment with effectively presenting the procedures, results, impressions, and recommendations to others in written form. Current concepts, practical considerations, current economic and health care climate, and legal and ethical matters will all come into play. There are numerous books available that emphasize the specifics of the actual diagnostic evaluation process or general professional writing. The goal of this book will be to focus on specifically writing the diagnostic evaluation. It is my hope that after reading this book, more clinicians will better appreciate the diagnostic writing process, become better and more accountable report writers, and view the diagnostic report not as a cumbersome necessity but as a palette on which to share their expertise, professional responsibility, and compassion with those who seek our services.

Understanding the Information in This Book

The goal of this textbook is to focus on the skills and processes necessary to successfully write clinical diagnostic speech and language evaluations. The ability to produce such a document is largely dependent upon the underlying knowledge and skills necessary to complete a thorough, evidence-based diagnostic evaluation for any number of speech and language disorders. The premise of the book is that the report writing process will follow a similar pathway regardless of the disorder and reason for referral. There are common aspects to completing an evaluation, and understanding the concepts involved in the process will facilitate the eventual documentation of the results in an evaluation. If one does not specifically focus on each individual disorder or problem and think that each report necessitates a different or unique style of writing, the result will be a more straightforward and less stressful way to present the results in a written format. The end result is to transfer what may be the results of hours and hours of testing and analysis and thought into a written format that the eventual end user of the report will appreciate and understand. This will ultimately benefit the individual who was seen for the evaluation and the report readers. The report is the only evidence of what was actually done.

It must be realized that it is impossible to deal with the report writing process without discussing and understanding the numerous techniques, skills, processes, and knowledge intricate to the actual assessment being conducted. The purpose of this book, however, is not to focus on the "how" to complete each specific evaluation but to focus on the "how" to think about and write the diagnostic evaluation. It is impossible to do this without discussing the assessment process. Any information presented regarding the evaluation process itself should be seen as being provided to increase evaluators' understanding of the elements involved in the evaluation, through a conceptual framework, with the ultimate goal of becoming a better report writer. Becoming a better evaluator of speech and language disorders will not necessarily make one a better, more skilled writer of reports or better at documentation. It is the opinion that becoming a better report writer requires thinking about one's writing and how to best transfer what was done in the evaluation to an evaluation report. This will conversely actually make one a better evaluator—learning to write reports with the thought that every line should be written with the thought that one day, never knowing when, the information contained in that report may be requested, called into question, subpoenaed, reviewed, or needed for a very specific purpose. The person's name at the bottom of the report will be the person ultimately responsible for the information contained in the document. With that in mind, thinking about what you will have to write and document will help guide what must be completed in the evaluation. After the individual to be evaluated leaves your office and the report is being generated, it is too late to realize the additional tests that you should have given, the subtest missed that eliminates the ability to correctly score a test, or the part of the oral examination that was left omitted or incomplete. The evaluation report can only be as complete, thorough, and accurate as the evaluation itself. Thus, what one writes is perhaps more important than what one does. It is often said and understood throughout the medical profession that "if it was not documented it was not done." Although this cliché is often used, it should serve as a guiding principle to one's report writing.

Some Terms That Must Be Clarified

Given the wide range of diagnostic disorders, ages, settings, types of assessments, numerous test instruments that are used, and the wide depth and breadth of the speech-language pathologist's role, it is impossible for the purposes of this text to restrict terminology to a single set of terms that could be used universally to explain what we do. This is an inherent difficulty within our profession, and it has always been that way. If one works in a school setting, the individuals we serve are our students; in a hospital, we work with our patients, and clients may come to our office. In a long-term care facility, we may see residents. We conduct evaluations, assessments, diagnostic evaluations, and consultations. We are speech-language pathologists, speech pathologists, therapists, and clinicians. These are terms that are sometimes used interchangeably, and their correct or incorrect use is still debated within our profession. The debate over terminology has even extended to disorders we treat in our professional discussions. One recent discussion is what exactly do we call the children we see with language disorders, specific language impairment, language delay, developmental language disorder, mixed receptive-expressive language disorder, or developmental language delay. There currently exists such a discussion within our literature with various individuals weighing in on the merits or problems with each of these terms.

For the purposes of this text, the terminology used at times may not be that critical to the discussion and therefore can be interchangeable and will not affect the overall meaning of the information provided. In other cases, the terminology used will be selected specifically as it relates more directly to the topic being presented. As is the case in our report writing, even the terminology and vocabulary must be carefully selected to maximize meaning, and understanding such will be the case throughout this text.

The chapters in this book, following some basic information, will follow the typical sequence of a typical diagnostic report. From the initial reason for the referral to the final recommendations and referrals, each chapter will present considerations, thoughts, and concepts on how to document each of the requisite steps in evaluating a patient or client.

The reader should think in terms of the broad assessment procedures used to evaluate communication disorders and, as importantly, the necessary documentation that must follow. They are integrated and inherently linked. While the knowledge and skills to assess each disorder are variable, documentation through report writing should be seen as a constant with far less variability. That is the goal of this book.

Diagnostic Report Writing
Initial Thoughts

As a speech-language pathologist, clinician, therapist, or whatever we choose to call ourselves, it is our responsibility to provide evidence-based assessment and treatment to those with a myriad of communication delays, disorders, and related difficulties. To do this, we must thoroughly question, evaluate, assess, test, judge, infer, analyze, and ultimately diagnose the nature and extent of the communication ability that our client or patient presents with. It may also require the recognition by the clinician that the presenting problem we are asked to evaluate is not actually within our realm. An individual's difficulty may be beyond our scope of practice, better treated by another professional (including another speech pathologist with more expertise in a given area), or in need of further evaluation by another discipline. This critical realization is part of the diagnostic process. The communication problem may defy a single diagnostic label, and sometimes it is only after weeks or months of working with a patient do we fully appreciate and understand all of the various contributing factors that will provide us with a conceptual understanding of what a particular disorder is and how to most effectively treat it.

Understanding the extent, severity, contributing factors, current levels of communicative function, summary, recommendations, test results, observations, informal assessments, standardized test results, and interpretations must all be cohesively condensed, integrated, and presented in a single document called the *diagnostic evaluation report*. It is the definitive outcome and documentation of how we will eventually share the critical information determined from the assessment process with

Blaustein, S. H. *Diagnostic Report Writing in Speech-Language Pathology:*
A Guide to Effective Communication (pp. 1-6).
© 2023 Taylor & Francis Group.

allied medical professionals, teachers, treating therapists, family members, referral sources, insurance companies, special education committees, and an ever-increasing array of individuals that will in some way have an impact on our clients' and patients' lives through the eventual intervention and related referral and placement processes. Levels of support, frequency and duration of therapeutic intervention, and financial determinations will all be based on information gleaned from our final diagnostic reports. Our evaluations may end up at impartial hearings for determination of eligibility for school-related services and reviewed for approval for insurance reimbursement based on plan criteria or in courts of law in a variety of proceedings, including medical malpractice or disability claims. These documents are important and relevant, have legal status, and are included and specified under various State Department of Education, Department of Health, Medicare, Medicaid, and many other regulations and guidelines. A written diagnostic evaluation report is not to be taken lightly and just done and "checked off" when the assessment process is completed.

Diagnostic reports are a measure of us as professionals; our signatures appear at the conclusion of each report. We bear ultimate responsibility for the contents of every report we write! Each written diagnostic report must be viewed considering an evaluator never knows what impact this document will ultimately have at some later point in time. One cannot predict which report will be subpoenaed, used at a hearing, requested by an insurance company, or questioned in any of a variety of matters. Each report must be written with all of these factors in mind. Most important, it is again emphasized that at the end of each report sits our signature. An accurate, well-written diagnostic report not only requires the knowledge and skills necessary to present one's work in written form, but at its core represents the sum total of one's diagnostic skill set effectively communicated to others. Evaluating a communication disorder is like completing a complex jigsaw puzzle. The various pieces must be identified, examined, viewed in a variety of ways, and eventually thoughtfully and meaningfully interconnected to fit and form a complete picture. The process must be respected. A missing piece, one incorrectly placed, or viewing the puzzle from the wrong angle will result in a distorted picture. In a diagnostic evaluation, incomplete data, insufficient or incorrect test results, or viewing the accumulated data with a preconceived, narrow, biased, or limited knowledge set will likely, if not certainly, result in an incomplete or incorrect diagnosis. Any resultant written diagnostic evaluation reflecting these errors will ultimately be detrimental to the care of the patient, can result in a flawed or limited treatment plan, can produce less than optimal recommendations, and perhaps skew appropriate referrals for additional consultation or care. Putting imprecise, flawed, or insufficient information into any document with our signature reflects on our professional integrity, can communicate erroneous information to others who are dependent on the evaluation, and ultimately may leave the evaluator liable for their findings. The diagnostic evaluation in its final written form will set the stage to indicate the need for no treatment, additional assessment, months of therapy, additional medical consults, and reactions from family members and those involved in a patient's care. Whatever may be communicated verbally, it is the written report that will bear the weight of accountability. The utmost thought and care must go into every written evaluation that is produced. It is too important to do any less. One should consistently be considering and prepared to answer the following questions as each report is generated:

1. Is every statement in this report factual?
2. Is the information presented in the clearest, most straightforward way?
3. Is the evaluation result as documented complete and thorough?
4. Is there any question of ambiguity or possible confusion?
5. If called upon to testify or support this document in any hearing, proceeding, or matter, can each and every statement, finding, result, and recommendation and referral be supported by evidence and clinical certainty?
6. Is this report sufficiently free of technical jargon to be understood and used by all who read it?
7. Has this report been read and edited for spelling, punctuation, and grammar?

8. Do the underlying notes, test data, authentic assessments, informal observations, case history, and all of the relevant information documented support the report as it stands, and is this information organized, correct, and available if needed? Is this report completely free of bias and fair?

9. Does the information and resultant conclusion contained in this report answer the diagnostic question provided in the reason for referral?

10. Will this report, including recommendations, best serve the client or patient with respect to the referring professionals, insurance companies, school districts, and so on?

If the answer to any of these questions is no, or questionable, more work is needed before a final draft of an evaluation should be signed and submitted. Every line written should be completed and edited with the question in mind, "If asked about this statement, in any way for any reason, can I support, justify, and explain it without question?"

A Question of Content

Current clinical practice and ethics dictate that we must practice our profession at the highest level of expertise, accountability, responsibility, and clinical awareness. Evidence-based practice (EBP) is widely recognized to be the cornerstone of our profession. As a result of current and potential future changes in national health care policies, greater use of the internet in transmission of personal health care information within the Health Insurance Portability and Accountability Act (HIPAA) guidelines, greater inclusion in the Medicare and Medicaid programs for speech-language pathology services, and greater competition for health care dollars from insurance companies, as providers, we must be at the top of our game to remain competitive and relevant. The documentation of our findings with respect to establishing initial needs and demonstrating rationales for ongoing treatment has never been more important. We are immersed in an alphabet of regulations and guidelines that have drastically changed laws for protecting individuals' health care rights. Concepts such as the Individuals with Disabilities Education Improvement Act (IDEA, 1975), Rehabilitation Act of 1973: Section 504, Family Educational Rights and Privacy Act (FERPA, 1974), No Child Left Behind (NCLB, 2002), Health Insurance Portability and Accountability Act (HIPAA, 1996), Committee on Special Education (CSE), Individualized Education Plan (IEP), Free and Appropriate Public Education (FAPE), and Americans with Disabilities Act (ADA, 1990) all have relevance for health care providers and educators across settings. Awareness of the contained rules, regulations, and requirements impacts speech-language pathologists. They specify types of information that may be required to be included in our documentation.

They also specify aspects of transfer of and access to information that clinicians also must be aware of. Clinicians must be well versed in each of these areas and more as they relate to their respective areas of practice. Evaluators must also be aware of ever-increasing layers of federal, state, local, and even school district rules and regulations that have increased paperwork, called for increased continuing education, and placed unprecedented demands on the time and resources of practicing speech-language pathologists nationwide. These requirements need to be fully understood, and the impact of these regulations will have to be considered in the diagnostic report. This will continue to be the state of practice and, if anything, become more of an issue in the future.

As a result of these demands, the American Speech-Language-Hearing Association (ASHA) has actively been providing extensive clinical practice guidelines and evidence maps, as well as promoting the concept of EBP among its membership (ASHA, 2004). Yet, to date, there has been little if any direct research or analysis paid to one of the most important aspects of our practice, the diagnostic evaluation report. While our graduate programs teach diagnostic report writing, there exists no one style, standard, requirement, or template specified by any association, organization, or regulatory body. While the information included in a diagnostic evaluation may generally be agreed upon based on requirements in our training and required information that must be documented is specified by numerous entities, there exists no one standard specified format to present this information. There are countless styles, formats, and templates and clinicians' personal feelings about the best way to present results and recommendations. Greater reliance on electronic medical records and increased availability of computer-assisted scoring for standardized tests and associated electronic medical record computer-generated reporting of results in narrative format will further increase the variety of documentation choices. There are numerous advantages to these newer documentation options in terms of efficiency and ease. There are also disadvantages in that clinicians must be careful not to overly rely on systems where data are simply uploaded and results and reports generated without a full understanding of the underlying principles and much-needed clinician analysis and opinion. Technology should be available to assist, not replace.

It Is Your Choice: Make It Right

In the absence of best practice guidelines and the limited availability of EBP data to support standardized guidelines to dictate the content, style, and form of each individual evaluation, it is left up to the experience, knowledge set, and judgment of each individual practitioner to generate individual diagnostic speech and language evaluation reports. The differences in diagnostic reports are further exacerbated by specific requirements necessitated by setting. This leads to the variations in style, form, and content we see in our professional diagnostic evaluation reports. A review of the literature in speech-language pathology yields scant, if any, research data dealing with effectiveness, utility, format, or reliability of diagnostic evaluations.

While every objective standardized assessment instrument we use contains data on the reliability and validity of the instrument (and much of this has lately been called into question), how the practitioner presents, synthesizes, and uses the data has received little attention. While a solo therapist in an employment setting or in private practice may have the latitude and flexibility to at least determine one's own representation of an acceptable and functional report, the wide variations, differences, diagnoses, test protocols, and ages of our populations served in a multitude of sites further serve to dilute a standard or cohesive format of any diagnostic evaluation document that we may wish to put forward as a unified profession. Realize that the reasons for variability in reports just mentioned may actually prohibit the ability to develop a more standardized report format. As professionals, we also wish to preserve our autonomy and ability to use our clinical opinion to produce the most correct and applicable final documentation possible. Recognizing these and other barriers to a more uniform diagnostic report for our profession, one must still accept and acknowledge the necessity to be aware of the basic requisite that must be present in every report we write.

Many times the eventual written document will reflect the mandates of the setting where one is employed. Thus, a hospital, rehabilitation center, school system, private practice group, or agency may each develop a specific template for what each report generated will include, specifying style, format, specific assessment instruments to be incorporated, and how results and recommendations are to be addressed. This makes sense as uniformity in documentation within each site must be maintained. Different sites will also be aware of the necessary documentation needs that must be included in each report based on needs for clients or patients qualifying for services or reimbursement. The variations in these reports can therefore be noticeably different from site to site. Lengthy overwritten narrative-style reports with every piece of information collected during the assessment can be the style of one institution contrasted against other sites that use limited outlines or checklist-style reports that contain just minimal data to support a diagnosis and provide sufficient information to be used to develop an adequate treatment plan. One may lend itself to including unnecessary, tangential, or irrelevant information while the latter may result in insufficient information to support placement or reimbursement. Ultimately, the evaluator and thus the report writer is hopefully left to the final decision as to what to include in the document they are producing within the constraints of the employment setting.

CONSIDERATIONS IN REPORT WRITING BY SETTING

The diagnostic report style called for is often determined by a variety of factors. These are often dictated by specific employment settings. Ideally, the requirements for a site's diagnostic report are current, evidence-based where applicable, and practical. It would also be preferable and logical that a speech-language pathologist had input into the development of the document used. Sometimes, however, this is not the case. There are reasons why a clinician may be asked to use template, form, or style of report with which they do not agree. These reasons may simply include traditional or outdated policies and procedures that may have not been routinely updated to reflect current trends and latest mandates, impacts from administrators who are not speech-language pathologists and whose considerations may reflect management, time or budgetary constraints, or creating formats for many staff over a period of time without cohesively maintaining appropriate current concepts. Whatever the reason, an evaluator working in an employment setting that fails to recognize accepted standards for completing and drafting a thorough, professional, and ethical evaluation report may be faced with a professional dilemma that might need to be addressed. The following specific guidelines should be considered and carefully weighed before accepting a position where a possibility exists that ASHA guidelines, ASHA Code of Ethics, federal or state regulations, professional standards, ethical integrity, or conflict of interest may fall into question regarding the diagnostic and reporting process.

1. Is there sufficient time, resources, adequate space, and a conducive environment available for testing? An evaluation cannot be rushed. The evaluator must be allowed enough time to obtain a history, observe behavior, properly complete all assessments, score and interpret results, and meet with clients or patients to provide feedback. If standardized test instruments are called for by the employer, they should be the most recent and revised editions in acceptable condition to be presented to individuals for whom they are intended.

2. Materials such as protective gloves, tongue depressors, cleansing agents, and sanitizing solutions are usually provided in employment settings. If not, it should be made clear whose responsibility and cost it will be to provide them.

3. A well-lit, well-ventilated, comfortable space free from distraction is needed to properly assess a patient or client. It should be properly furnished. Hallways, shared spaces, noisy classrooms, and similar environments can negatively impact an accurate assessment.

4. If the report is to be typed, mailed, copied, emailed, or transferred, is there sufficient clerical staff to assist in such tasks? If not, on whose shoulders do these responsibilities fall? Is time allotted, and is there additional compensation if responsibility falls on the evaluator?

5. Many contract agencies currently determine a rate for a set amount of time to complete an evaluation. Time to score tests, analyze, write, and prepare the diagnostic report is done on the evaluator's time beyond the actual client or patient contact hours and may or may not be included in the evaluation reimbursement rate. This must always be clarified.

6. Is the content of the evaluation set by the employer or the evaluator? In some instances, an evaluation may be limited to a specific test or set of tests prescribed by the employer. Is this battery broad enough? Can additional or extended testing be completed? Whose decision is this, and is there a variety of additional appropriate assessment materials available suitable to the population served by the setting?

7. Is there freedom to express proper results, conclusions, and recommendations without limitations, unreasonable caps on frequencies, and durations of treatments? Is the patient or client free to seek services elsewhere and free and encouraged to obtain second opinions, or does the facility encourage individuals to obtain their therapies at their own site, creating possible unreasonable appearing conflicts of interest?

8. Will final diagnostic reports be supervised, edited, cosigned, or in any other way influenced by others at the site? While these influences are encouraged or even required for Clinical Fellowship therapists or those with less experience with a particular disorder, unreasonable, unprofessional, unethical, or overreaching demands or requests for changes to an evaluation can constrain or compromise the integrity of any clinician if unduly imposed.

It can thus be seen that long before one sits down to prepare the final diagnostic report, there are numerous considerations, responsibilities, and details that must be considered. The challenge to accept the role of evaluating a communication disorder and then to place those findings into a final diagnostic report can have broad and far-reaching impact. It is a task that is not to be taken lightly.

REFERENCE

American Speech-Language-Hearing Association. (2004). *Preferred practice patterns for the profession of speech-language pathology.* https://www.asha.org/policy/pp2004-00191

Some Notes on Report Writing Style

There are many books available on clinical documentation and professional report writing. These texts often contain information on basic writing skills, American Psychological Association (APA; 2020) style, grammar, and punctuation. By the time a professional is in a position to be conducting a speech and language evaluation, it should be assumed that competent writing skills have been mastered and that final evaluation reports should be carefully proofread for these elements. Basics of writing as part of the report writing process will not be reviewed in this book. There are, however, a number of common errors that frequently occur when beginning to write diagnostic reports that will be discussed. These are not related to the basic grammar and punctuation errors one should already be aware of. What does not come naturally and what must be learned is clinical report writing style and content. The subtle, specific, and unique presentation of information that is needed to generate competent clinical reports will be highlighted as part of the explanations and descriptions of diagnostic report content. This style of writing is new to students, has its own rules and elements to consider, and requires practice. Having the basic writing essentials that will underlie these elements is necessary and helpful. If a review is needed, it is suggested that one become familiar with the fundamentals of writing in one of the many sources readily available.

Blaustein, S. H. *Diagnostic Report Writing in Speech–Language Pathology: A Guide to Effective Communication* (pp. 7-12).
© 2023 Taylor & Francis Group.

It goes without saying that any report that bears one's signature should contain accurate spelling, punctuation, grammar, formatting, and all the core writing characteristics that are expected from a professional in any written document. Once a written report leaves the professional's office, it is in another's hands, read by many, and scrutinized, and any errors in basic writing skills will reflect back on the competence of the evaluator and the quality of the report. Once words are permanently put to paper or digitally produced, no one will correct them for the evaluator, but they will certainly be noticed.

In reading and reviewing evaluation reports from students and professionals, common errors are frequently seen in speech and language evaluations that are not necessarily related to simple spelling or punctuation. These are presented here for review and should be considered when producing and finalizing a written speech and language evaluation. The following points are based on the author's experience in working with hundreds of students in developing professional report writing style and in reading and producing countless professional reports. The following factors should be kept in mind:

1. **The use of abbreviations for tests, diagnoses, and procedures should be carefully monitored.**

It has become common for speech-language pathologists, as well as many other professionals, to use abbreviations frequently in our written and verbal communications. Look at the huge number of abbreviations and initials that are now accepted as commonplace as a result of texting and social media. It has become so common to use abbreviations for tests that the abbreviations have become acronyms that seem to have replaced the names of the actual tests, diagnoses, or procedures. Initials have made their way into written reports and conversations with the actual label becoming minimized or even eliminated. For example, the Clinical Evaluation of Language Fundamentals-5 (Wiig et al., 2013), a common, often-used test in its fifth edition, is often referred to as the CELF-5. Autism spectrum disorder is now ASD, and augmentative and alternative communication is more commonly referred to as AAC. The Goldman Fristoe Test of Articulation-3 (Goldman & Fristoe, 2015), a frequently used test that has been around for 40 years, has become the GFTA and is actually frequently referred to by the sound of the four letters "Gifta." Our professional title of speech-language pathologist is frequently referred to as the "SLP" and these initials have evolved to a point where they are now frequently used in our reports and professional documents. It is surprising to realize how many graduate students and even professionals cannot state what many of the commonly used initials stand for.

While those in the field of speech-language pathology may be familiar with these abbreviations and understand their meaning, most others will not. An evaluator should be certain that when referring to any component that will later be represented by initials in a document that the component be first correctly and clearly labeled in the initial reference. In a first reference to an item to be later abbreviated, such as a test, the item should be correctly documented, such as the CELF-5. The reader will later recognize what the abbreviation utilized represents. Childhood apraxia of speech has now generally been accepted as CAS to those familiar with this speech disorder. It should be initially referenced in a report as "The client is being seen to rule out suspected childhood apraxia of speech (CAS)." Students and professionals have become so accustomed to the use of initials and acronyms that their use is often not questioned.

2. **Use initials for client's or patient's names only when and where appropriate.**

Just as it has become common for students and clinicians new to the field to frequently rely on initials for tests, disorders, and procedures, it has also become common for some clinicians to use initials when referring to clients or patients. There is a reason for the use of initials in place of names, but that reason must be understood to enable the evaluator to determine when and where to use initials.

Patient and client confidentiality is a serious legal and ethical concern. While privacy has always been an issue in the health profession, with the passing of the Health Insurance Portability and Accountability Act (HIPAA, 1996), confidentiality has become an essential element within health care professions. The training and use of HIPAA is of utmost importance, and violations and breaches of HIPAA compliance can carry serious consequences.

The use of initials for an individual who is receiving health care services, especially during student training, stems from protecting the confidentiality of the individual being evaluated or receiving intervention at certain times. When sharing reports with other students, with information transferring back and forth to supervisors and professors, and with reports and information perhaps, and not appropriately, being taken outside of the clinic or therapy environment, an individual's right to privacy is compromised. Using initials or even coding of patients using letters or numbers has become part of student training often mandated by clinical supervisors. The reason this is done has not, however, become universally understood, and after a clinician's training has been completed, reports may continue to be written utilizing the patient's initials in the body of the report. This "habit" extends to formal written documents and correspondence when there is no longer a need to do so. Once a final document is generated, it is common sense and required that an individual's actual name and other identifying information, such as date of birth, address, or workplace, be included as a necessary part of maintaining an individual's medical records. It is eventually necessary to correct and complete records for our clients and patients. Once that transition occurs, from initials to the correct identity, there are numerous extra layers of protection for these records containing an individual's personal information. These methods are well specified, required, monitored, and carefully addressed across all medical and health-related settings. Locked files, HIPAA compliance protocols, computer security through user identification and passwords, signed release forms, and other methods are in place to protect the client's and patient's information. Even methods of reporting "breaches" in patient confidentiality need to be in place. Individuals need to be aware of the when, why, and how of using personal identifying information. For example, if a report were to be used in teaching, educational setting, or publication, then the personal information may be again removed from the original document. The report is redacted to remove all identifying information, and appropriate permissions and releases should be obtained before using the patient's evaluation and diagnostic information in any way. Initials in a final written report that is sent to an authorized and appropriate recipient where the proper releases have been obtained need not be used.

3. **Be careful of the overuse of professional "jargon."**

Every profession has its own specialized and technical vocabulary. The profession of speech-language pathology is no different. Speech-language pathologists assess communication skills, diagnose disorders, establish intervention plans, and engage in numerous related professional and interprofessional activities. In our work, we have understandably developed, normalized, and used a specific professional lexicon that describes, specifies, labels, and indicates what we evaluate, analyze, and report. Much of this information, by its nature, must appear in our final written speech and language evaluation. It must be considered that while other speech-language pathologists will often use and read our reports, perhaps the majority of eventual readers and users of our assessments will not be speech-language pathologists. They are the ones who would be most familiar with our technical specialized terminology. Physicians, related health providers, psychologists, family members, teachers, tutors, administrators, and reviewers for third-party payers are but a few of the related persons who will have a need to use our reports for a variety of reasons. What we finally explain, assess, diagnose, and document and the eventual recommendations and referrals we provide must have meaning and be able to be understood by those outside of our field. Obviously, as in other professions, we cannot entirely escape our unique vocabulary. Consideration, therefore, must be given, when needed, for a few additional words of explanation to clarify terminology or vocabulary that would not be understood by those outside of our profession.

Diadochokinetic rates, phonological processes, and cluttering are but a few examples of terms known to those who are familiar with speech and language assessments but will have no meaning to those who have not encountered these terms previously. When too many of these terms are placed in our reports and documents, it adds an unfamiliar lexical density that could make it difficult for a parent, pediatrician, or reviewer to understand the precise nature of the difficulties their child or patient might actually be experiencing. It is important, therefore, to not only read one's report from our own professional perspective but give thought to the individual at a committee on preschool education meeting or in a skilled nursing facility who must make decisions regarding necessity for placements and intervention based on a report they are attempting to decipher.

4. **Be clear and concise and avoid overexplaining.**

Speech and language evaluation reports often include unneeded words, descriptions, phrasing, explanation, and detail that do not necessarily provide any additional meaning, information, or content to the report but transform what should be a professional clinical summary into a clinical "story." It is not necessary to begin a sentence with "In reference to the birth history. . ." or "Regarding the patient's articulation. . ." It is enough to state "Birth history was unremarkable as reported" or "Articulation is characterized by numerous substitutions and omissions." Similarly, it is not necessary to describe in detail an evident process such as obtaining a case history. For example, it is not necessary, efficient, or relevant to state in a written report that "The clinician asked Jason's mother at what age first words emerged," and then to provide an answer such as "Jason's mother reported that first words emerged at approximately 15 months of age." Simply stating "Onset of first words occurred at 15 months of age, as reported." The meaning is certainly the same, and once the informant has been indicated in the report, it is clear where the information was obtained.

The inclusion of wordy, descriptive, obvious information takes time to document, adds length to reports, adds little if any additional information, and adds time to the individual eventually reading the final document. Learning how to complete a condensed, concise, and accurate report is difficult, but once mastered through practice and guidance, it results in a more professional and clinically appropriate result.

5. **Be clear in referencing information and the use of pronouns.**

It is important when attempting to write concisely to also write clearly and accurately. A basic rule of speaking and writing is that before a pronoun is used, the referent (person, object, place) is first clearly labeled, defined, or identified prior to using a pronoun in its place. In the statement "Vegetables are healthy, and you should eat them every day," the pronoun "them" clearly refers to the vegetables referenced in the beginning of the sentence. Imagine the confusion to read "They are healthy if you eat them every day." Failure to follow simple rules of proper referencing will lead to confusion and misinterpretations in clinical report writing. This may happen in any style of writing or speaking, but when it occurs in a clinical report, which frequently happens as one develops clinical style, it can be a problem. To state, "John Smith and his son Ted Smith served as informants. He reported difficulty with memory which began 6 months ago." It becomes unclear whether John or his son provided the information, as they were both referenced in the initial statement equally. Similarly, in a statement such as "The Receptive One-Word Picture Vocabulary Test-4 and Expressive Vocabulary Test-2 were administered. It indicated reduced single-item vocabulary." The question can be raised, does the "it" in the second sentence refer to the administration and results of both tests or just one of the two. If it is just one of the two, which one is it? The results, thoughts, ideas, and conceptualizations in an evaluating clinician's mind must clearly and accurately be put to paper or digitally stored, and this information must translate clearly and accurately to the reader. Simple grammatical errors such as these can lead to misinformation.

In a discussion of pronouns, it should be mentioned that clinical reports are not written in the first person but in the third. This may seem obvious, but it is a very basic premise in report writing that is still ignored in early attempts in documentation and report writing. A final written evaluation should not contain a sentence such as, "I asked the patient to read the rainbow passage to me" but rather be documented as, "Patient was asked to read the rainbow passage." As obvious as this may seem, it occurs in reports and is therefore worth noting. An evaluator should also consider awareness of gender diversity in selecting and using personal pronouns. It is currently suggested in many health care settings that evaluators, as well as other professionals, ask individuals for their pronouns as part of the intake process.

Table 2-1
Common Errors to Avoid in Clinical Documentation
• Abbreviations should be used carefully, and the underlying meanings must be clearly stated before the use of an abbreviation.
• Initials for clients or patients should be used when and where appropriate.
• Professional jargon should be used carefully and explained where necessary.
• Clear and concise descriptions and explanations should be used over lengthy descriptions and unnecessary phrasing and syntax.
• The use of pronouns and referencing information should be clear in reports.
• Avoid subjective vocabulary use in clinical documentation when not needed.

6. **Avoid unneeded subjective vocabulary.**

Words have meaning. Subtle shades of differences in a word can nuance a reader's interpretation and understanding. Unless there is a reason not to, when an informant is providing a case history, the evaluator should choose neutral verbs to indicate the reporting of the information. The use of words such as the informant "stated, reported, indicated, or informed" that they were having difficulty with communication at work conveys an unbiased description of what the information was provided. The use of the neutral verbs signifies a simple transfer of information. A different meaning is inferred if the patient "admitted, lamented, exclaimed, or regretted" that they were having difficulty with communication at work. The substitution of words that may be emotionally laden or contain a different shade of meaning than a simple report should be carefully considered. Of course, if the informant actually states, "I admit that work has been difficult," the word "admit" should be used if the evaluator determines it is important to place that statement in the report. But the word "admit" should be placed in direct quotes as an indication that it was actually spoken by the patient. This type of precise reporting clarifies the documentation for both the reader and the evaluator. If a question arises later on as to the source of specific information, which can be months or years later, it makes it specifically clear that the patient reported the information as an "admission" rather than the statement being an interpretation as subjectively understood by the evaluator.

Similar care should be given to all vocabulary used in clinical documentation when reporting results, events experienced, symptoms, and so on. A child should be reported as "having frequent middle ear infections" rather than stating a child "suffered frequent ear infections." The use of "had" vs. "suffered" is a more neutral word with less emotional inferencing. There are frequent examples of this type of careful selection of semantic content. An "active" adolescent is not necessarily "hyperactive" and a patient who may refuse to complete a task is not automatically "oppositional." Care must be taken that vocabulary is selected that accurately and objectively reports events rather than having them interpreted subjectively through the evaluator's determination. Of course, an examiner may choose a specific word for a specific reason and the nuanced meaning may be a clear intent of the evaluator, but the overall concept here is that vocabulary makes a difference.

Table 2-1 summarizes the common errors to avoid in report writing. It can be used as a quick checklist and reminder prior to submitting clinical reports. It is by no means a complete list of all of the possible errors that may occur in a report. All clinical reports should be clearly proofread.

REFERENCES

American Psychological Association. (2020). *Publication manual of the American Psychological Association* (7th ed.). American Psychological Association.

Goldman, R., & Fristoe, M. (2015). *Goldman-Fristoe test of articulation 3* (3rd ed.). Pearson.

Health Insurance Portability and Accountability Act of 1996 (1996; 104th Congress H.R. 3103). HIPAA; Pub. L. 104–191, 110 Stat. 1936. https:govtrack.us/congress/bills/104/hr3103

Wiig, E., Semel, E., & Secord, W. (2013). *Clinical evaluation of language fundamentals, 5th ed. (CELF-5).* NCS Pearson, USA.

Ethics, Fairness, and Law
An Important Trio

There is no one standard format or style as to how to write a speech and language evaluation report. There are, however, certain responsibilities, foundations, concepts, and principles that must be adhered to. These responsibilities occur on many levels and are specified in numerous ways originating in a number of places. This chapter will present basic considerations that underlie written diagnostic reports. In viewing the report writing process in a conceptual framework, this is a good place to begin. Basic principles of report writing should carry through every diagnostic evaluation completed and will eventually become automatic once practiced and learned. The reasons for a particular evaluation, the referral source, tests selected, results, diagnosis, and recommendations will vary from assessment to assessment and evaluation site to evaluation site. The principles presented here will not vary. Basic issues of documentation, ethics, fairness, and law must carry into every written report. The principles to be discussed here are core to professional documentation and should also be kept in mind for all professional writing one produces, including progress notes, session notes, correspondence, and so on. These principles are in place to protect us, protect our patients and clients, ensure integrity, guarantee equity, and demonstrate fairness in evaluating the individuals we serve. They will serve as a lens through which our work can be viewed if ever called into question. Our written diagnostic evaluations are legal documents that must be preserved in a set manner for specified time periods and are used for many critical purposes.

Blaustein, S. H. *Diagnostic Report Writing in Speech–Language Pathology:*
A Guide to Effective Communication (pp. 13-19).
© 2023 Taylor & Francis Group.

TABLE 3-1	
Helpful American Speech-Language-Hearing Association Resources for Documentation	
ASHA SITE	**CONTENT**
Practice Portal	Guides evidence-based decision making on clinical and professional issues
Billing and Reimbursement	Information on coding, Medicare, Medicaid, and private health plans
Ethics	Code of Ethics, promote standards of integrity and ethics
Interprofessional Practice	Information on collaboration to improve clinical outcomes
Evidence-Based Practice	Latest summarized evidence on service delivery
Multicultural Resources	Information on cultural and linguistic diversity
Documentation Templates	Examples of various templates to be used or modified; not required by ASHA
Professional Issues	Documentation in health care, documentation in schools
Preferred Practice Patterns	A guide to promote quality patient care, including documentation in more than 45 areas of assessment and intervention
ASHA Policy Documents	Written by and for ASHA members and approved by governance; includes scope of practice, guidelines, and position statements to promote best standards in the profession

DOCUMENTATION

The American Speech-Language-Hearing Association (ASHA) serves many functions for its members and the public, including providing accreditation for clinical programs serving clients and patients, accrediting our educational training programs through the Council on Academic Accreditation, and certifying speech-language pathologists for entry into the Clinical Fellowship to eventually awarding the ASHA Certificate of Clinical Competence. Through a strict, nationally recognized program of requirements, standards, site visits, continuing education programs, position papers, and publications, ASHA advocates for our profession, increases public knowledge, and represents members and the individuals we serve to maintain the highest level of care for individuals with communication and swallowing challenges. What, then, does ASHA say about documenting and writing evaluation reports?

ASHA has an extensive website (www.asha.org) with a wide depth and breadth of information for its members and consumers. The reader is encouraged to use this valuable information resource to locate specific detailed information on documentation and links to important sources covering this critical area. Table 3-1 presents a list of some key areas that can be found on the ASHA website that clinicians should be aware of and reference as needed. The ASHA Practice Portal is a recommended place to start.

In general, ASHA reiterates the often heard, taught, and repeated mantra in medical and educational settings, "If it was not documented, it was not done!" In discussing "how" to document, we begin to see why students, in particular, Clinical Fellowship candidates and even experienced professionals, may puzzle over how to best present the results of a diagnostic speech and language evaluation. Note the following statement regarding documentation that ASHA presents in the "Documentation in Health Care Settings" section of the Practice Portal (ASHA, n.d.):

Because of the diversity of settings and payers, ASHA does not dictate a single format or time frame for documentation. State or federal agencies governing health care or licensure for speech-language pathologists may have specific requirements; if those requirements are more stringent, they supersede requirements of facilities, payers, and employment contractors.

This is logical, clear, and makes sense. We clearly must document our work, but the "what" to document is much less clear. In preparing our reports, we must be aware of who the referral source is, who will be funding the services, and who will be reviewing any requests associated with our patient and the information required. It would be impossible to set a specific set of criteria for every evaluation and subsequent report we generate. What do we do, then? One possible answer is to provide a general set of guidelines specifying areas to include in our reports. If we limit our focus to evaluation and diagnosis in medical settings, then we can consider following guidelines as specified by ASHA:

"Evaluation Report: The evaluation report typically is a summary of the evaluation process, any resulting diagnosis, and a plan for service and may include the following elements:

- reasons for referral;
- case history, including prior level of function, medical complexities, and comorbidities;
- review of auditory, visual, motor, and cognitive status;
- standardized and/or nonstandardized methods of evaluation;
- diagnosis;
- analysis and integration of information to develop prognosis, including outcomes measures and projected outcomes; and
- recommendations, including
  ○ referrals to other professionals as needed,
  ○ plan of care—
    ▪ treatment amount, frequency, and duration;
    ▪ long- and short-term functional goals (see International Classification of Functioning, Disability and Health framework)."

Thus, we have an outline of elements to be included in an evaluation, but a specific format for presentation, questions for a case history, and selection of assessment measures are left to the individual practitioner. Further direction for critical elements for an evaluation may be found on ASHA's website when searching "Preferred Practice Patterns—Assessment," where a more specific description of elements may be found classified by diagnosis. Thus, an evaluator should be fully aware of the elements that constitute an evaluation, but less guidance and structure are provided regarding how to gather this information and, just as important, how to present it. Given the inherent nature of the vast variety of diagnoses, settings, and referral sources we encounter as a profession, this makes sense. It is also why evaluators sometimes struggle with producing appropriate and useful reports.

Flexibility, knowledge, and skill must be used in completing our evaluations and producing the eventual written report. If we view the process conceptually and understand the "what" we need to include in an evaluation, we should then be able to similarly deduce "what" we need to document. One follows the other.

To further illustrate the idea of having the concept of knowing what to do will lead to what to present, consider ASHA's statement on "Documentation in Educational Settings." It is not unlike documentation in medical settings. The variance by setting is again stated as a factor in our documentation.

Education Settings: Documentation formats vary among education systems, and ASHA does not dictate a single format or time frame. State or federal agencies governing schools, Medicaid reimbursement, or audiology and speech-language pathology regulations may have specific requirements for documentation. Any documentation must meet state and federal agency requirements. School districts, payers, or employment contractors may have additional requirements.

It is important that the information presented here be understood by the speech-language pathologist completing the assessment and documenting it. We have general guidelines that must consistently transfer across our reports. The relative weight of this information, the amount of information, how the information is collected, and, most importantly, how this information is analyzed, interpreted, and presented are variable. It is dependent on the specific needs of the client or patient, setting, who is the eventual user of the report, and what information is needed. Understanding this concept will make report writing less ambiguous, difficult, and confusing. One size does not fit all.

Ethics

It goes without saying that any individual providing evaluation or treatment service to a person with a communication or swallowing disorder will demonstrate ethical and professional behavior and hold themselves and others to the highest standards. To ensure that there is an agreed upon specification of what constitutes ethical and professional behavior, ASHA maintains and regularly reviews and updates a Code of Ethics. They are described on ASHA's website as follows:

> The ASHA Code of Ethics is a framework and focused guide for professionals in support of day-to-day decision making related to professional conduct. The Code is partly obligatory and disciplinary and partly aspirational and descriptive in that it defines the professional's role. The Code educates professionals in the discipline, as well as students, other professionals, and the public, regarding ethical principles and standards that direct professional conduct. (ASHA, 2016)

Individuals found in violation of the Code of Ethics are liable for a variety of consequences that may be imposed following a review by the Board of Ethics. Individuals may be reported by other professionals, clients, patients, the public, or self-report. Actions imposed can range from censure to revocation of certification for a period of time up to and including life based on the severity of the infraction.

There are stated standards that are organized in four broad areas. The reader is directed to the ASHA website for the complete list. Five specific ASHA Code of Ethics standards have been selected that pertain more directly to the assessment and evaluation process and have been selected by the author to illustrate examples of the Code of Ethics that are most relevant to this text. It is strongly advised that any practicing speech-language pathologist familiarize themselves with the complete document. The standards selected concern use of independent and evidence-based judgment, confidentiality, timeliness and accuracy of records, scope of practice, and misrepresenting diagnostic and other information. The Roman numerals and letters refer to the ASHA Code of Ethics guideline.

I. (M) Individuals who hold the Certificate of Clinical Competence shall use independent and evidence-based clinical judgment, keeping paramount the best interests of those being served.

(O) Individuals shall protect the confidentiality and security of records of professional services provided, research and scholarly activities conducted, and products dispensed. Access to these records shall be allowed only when doing so is necessary to protect the welfare of the person or of the community, is legally authorized, or is otherwise required by law.

(Q) Individuals shall maintain timely records and accurately record and bill for services provided and products dispensed and shall not misrepresent services provided, products dispensed, or research and scholarly activities conducted.

II. (A) Individuals who hold the Certificate of Clinical Competence shall engage in only those aspects of the professions that are within the scope of their professional practice and competence, considering their certification status, education, training, and experience.

III. (C) Individuals shall not misrepresent research and scholarly activities, diagnostic information, services provided, results of services provided, products dispensed, or the effects of products dispensed.

Ethical behavior is and has always been of the utmost concern to professionals and the consumers we serve. That is why descriptions of professional ethical behavior do not stop with ASHA. Each state licensing board, state or local professional organizations, and individual employment settings, such as universities, medical settings, and school districts, may have their own codes, regulations, rules, or standards that professionals must also be aware of. The importance of ethics was further highlighted when ASHA specified that as of 2020, all members must complete at least three continuing education credits in the area of ethics.

While the idea of respecting diversity, equity, and inclusion is relevant to many areas of documenting our assessments, placing the discussion within the ethics section seems quite appropriate. It is essential that all clinicians demonstrate cultural competence and provide culturally responsive services in every aspect of what we do as professionals. From the initial contact with our clients, patients, and those who support them through the clinician's assessment, diagnosis, interventions, counseling, recommendations and referrals, cultural and linguistic competence must be at the forefront of our interactions. It is essential that awareness and respect for cultural and linguistic diversity be evident in all of our clinical documentation including our diagnostic evaluation reports. The knowledge and skills that lead to evidence-based and culturally aware assessments must be embedded into the reporting and documentation of our evaluations.

Clinicians must be well versed in areas including multicultural policies and procedures, multicultural and multilingual issues, culturally and linguistically diverse populations, gender diversity, equity, inclusion, and within all of the related areas of knowledge and skills required for clinical practice. The words we select, how we use them, and, for the purposes of this book, how we write them are as critical as the services we provide. The incorrect use of a pronoun or inappropriate phrase in a report can make a great deal of difference. The reader is directed to the ASHA website (www.asha.org) as a valuable resource for culturally and linguistically diverse and multicultural and multilingual issues.

FAIRNESS

Without sitting down to write one's first evaluation report, the amount of information that is required to consider in documentation is significant. Additional attention must be given to the Code of Fair Testing Practices in Education. This document, prepared by the Joint Committee on Testing Practices (2004), delineates aspects of fairness in testing that must be considered by both test developers and test users. The Code, endorsed by seven professional organizations, including ASHA and the American Psychological Association, presents a comprehensive series of guidelines to cover the educational use of testing used for assessment, diagnosis, and placement. The following description is contained in the code: "The Code of Fair Testing Practices in Education is a guide for professionals in fulfilling their obligation to provide and use tests that are fair to all test takers regardless of age, gender, disability, race, ethnicity, national origin, religion, sexual orientation, linguistic background, or other personal characteristics. Fairness is a primary consideration in all aspects of testing."

The Code is divided into four areas that include (A) Development and Assessment, (B) Administration and Scoring, (C) Reporting and Interpreting, and (D) Informing Test Takers. The areas are further divided into two areas that include statements for test developers and test users. For the purposes of this text, the author has selected to reference Section (C) with "information for test users concerning reporting and interpreting test results" as presented in the Code of Fair Practices in Education (Section C, 1–8).

C-1. Interpret the meaning of the test results, taking into account the nature of the content, norms, or comparison groups, other technical evidence, and benefits and limitations of test results.

C-2. Interpret test results from modified test or test administration procedures in view of the impact those modifications may have had on test results.

C-3. Avoid using tests for purposes other than those recommended by the test developer unless there is evidence to support the intended use or interpretation.

C-4. Review the procedures for setting performance standards or passing scores. Avoid using stigmatizing labels.

C-5. Avoid using a single test score as the sole determinant of decisions about test takers. Interpret test scores in conjunction with other information about individuals.

C-6. State the intended interpretation and use of test results for groups of test takers. Avoid grouping test results for purposes not specifically recommended by the test developer unless evidence is obtained to support the intended use. Report procedures that were followed in determining who were and who were not included in the groups being compared and describe factors that might influence the interpretation of results.

C-7. Communicate test results in a timely fashion and in a manner that is understood by the test taker.

C-8. Develop and implement procedures for monitoring test use, including consistency with the intended purposes of the test.

LAW

While ASHA provides members with guidelines, recommendations, best practices, and position statements, these are not legislated. Violation of certain ASHA guidelines or Code of Ethics violations can result in suspension or revocation of a clinician's membership, impacting ability to practice; these are not criminal penalties. There are, however, regulations, requirements, statutes, and mandates that are legislated that must be followed. Many relate directly to components of report writing and documentation. Most, if not all, speech pathologists are now required to be licensed by the state(s) in which they practice. They set requirements, guidelines, and regulations in addition to those mandated by local and state legislators. Evaluators must be aware of and abide by these mandates.

For example, recently, as a result of COVID-19 and the ensuing pandemic, individuals across the country were forced to relocate. Many individuals receiving speech and language therapy services relocated to other states. Clients requested that therapies continue via telepractice. This created a dilemma that was realized by the states and ASHA. It became clear speech clinicians could only practice in the state in which they were licensed. As a result, states set emergency guidelines allowing out-of-state practitioners to engage in telepractice without being licensed under specified, qualified conditions. That varied from state to state. Clinicians needed to be keenly aware of each state's regulations in which they chose to continue to provide interventions. ASHA facilitated and enabled the process by publishing regulations by state.

When documenting evaluation results through written reports, there are numerous legal requirements, statutes, and regulations that must be considered. These include regulations governing sharing information, such as those specified under the Health Insurance Portability and Accountability Act (1996) and the Family Educational Rights and Privacy Act (1974). State regulations also may specify how long medical records must be maintained and provisions for allowing a client's or patient's access to their records. Federal mandates, including the Individuals with Disabilities Education Improvement Act (1975) and Section 504 of the Rehabilitation Act of 1973 contain further provisions that speech-language pathologists must be aware of. Medicare and Medicaid are additional programs that have a significant number of regulations and requirements embedded within their programs that must be followed by speech-language pathologists. These will further be discussed in Chapter 10.

The intended point here is that we do not practice in a vacuum, and choices we make in documentation must be based not only on ethics, knowledge, skills, and fairness, but also on law. Speech-language pathologists in their work are surrounded by a sea of initials representing numerous regulations and guidelines that must be considered in documentation. Table 3-2 summarizes a list of some

TABLE 3-2	Ten Key Abbreviations for Speech-Language Pathologists to Know
ADA	Americans with Disabilities Act (https://www.ada.gov/ada_fed_resources.htm)
CMS	Centers for Medicare & Medicaid Services (https://www.cms.gov/)
EI	Early Intervention Program for Infants and Toddlers (https://www2.ed.gov/programs/osepeip/legislation.html)
FAPE	Free and Appropriate Public Education (https://www2.ed.gov/about/offices/list/ocr/docs/edlite-FAPE504.html)
FERPA	Family Education Rights and Privacy Act 1974 (https://www2.ed.gov/about/offices/list/ocr/docs/edlite-FAPE504.html)
HIPAA	Health Insurance Portability and Accountability Act (https://www.cdc.gov/phlp/publications/topic/hipaa.html)
IDEA	Individuals with Disabilities Education Act 2004 (https://sites.ed.gov/idea/about-idea/)
IEP	Individualized Education Plan (https://www2.ed.gov/parents/needs/speced/iepguide/index.html)
LRE	Least Restrictive Environment (https://sites.ed.gov/idea/regs/b/b/300.114)
504 Plan	Part of Rehabilitation Act of 1973 (https://www2.ed.gov/about/offices/list/ocr/504faq.html)

of the ones more frequently used and should, at a minimum, be understood in our documentation. We must always be aware of, and practice under, the umbrella of federal state and local requirements. These must be respected and adhered to. Failure to do so may not only result in consequences, including suspension or loss of one's license and certification, but fines can also be imposed. More severe violations, such as fraud, have resulted in imprisonment.

In summary, ethics, fairness, and law are three key principles that must be respected in the practice of speech-language pathology. An important and critical aspect of this practice is documentation. In any question or violation under scrutiny, our records, reports, and notes will certainly be reviewed. These considerations cannot be ignored.

REFERENCES

American Speech-Language-Hearing Association. (n.d.). *Module 3: Documentation of SLP services in different settings.* http://www.ash.org/Practice/reimbursement/Module-Three-Transcript/

American Speech-Language-Hearing Association. (2016). *Code of ethics.* www.asha.org/policy/

Joint Committee on Testing Practices. (2004). *Code of fair testing practices in education.* https://www.academia.edu/2950725/Code_of_Fair_Testing_Practices_in_Education

A Reason for the Reason for Referral and a Case for the Case History

If a clinician begins to understand the idea that a written diagnostic evaluation report must be produced following each and every evaluation completed, then one can begin to realize that the report is just one more part of the process. The steps in actually conducting a speech and language evaluation follow a series of sequenced logical procedures and tasks. The report writing process must therefore follow those same sequenced steps. Conducting a speech and language evaluation consists of ordered tasks with a learned and logical progression. It begins with the reason for the referral and progresses to the determination of recommendations and referrals. The specific questions to be asked, assessment instruments, and types of informal authentic tasks will vary by diagnosis, but the overriding task of evaluation will involve the same core procedures that must be done to gain the necessary information to arrive at a summary and conclusion. The written report that follows the evaluation should be thought of similarly. It will mirror, in written form, the actual evaluation as it was conducted. The final written report can then be viewed conceptually as a series of written descriptions of the processes and procedures completed during the assessment with varying content based on the nature of the disorder being assessed. Each and every evaluation will begin with a reason for the referral. A statement regarding the reason for the referral of an individual is therefore a logical place to start the written report. This is also, at times, referred to in a report as the "statement of the problem."

Blaustein, S. H. *Diagnostic Report Writing in Speech–Language Pathology: A Guide to Effective Communication* (pp. 21-29). © 2023 Taylor & Francis Group.

Initially, stating the reason(s) that an evaluation is being performed in the report serves a number of important functions for both the reader and the evaluator. For the reader, it orients the eventual end user of the report to the basic reason an evaluation was conducted. It will specify who referred the individual and is requesting the evaluation, who accompanied the individual to the evaluation, and, most importantly, why the evaluation is being conducted. Specific problems to be addressed during the evaluation may also be stated. These will become the issues and questions that must eventually be answered at the conclusion of the report by the evaluator.

In some instances, the individual being evaluated will be seen after having received a previous established diagnosis that will be helpful to be aware of. It will often be provided by the individual making the referral for the speech and language evaluation and should be documented along with the reason for the speech and language assessment being requested. Many diseases, disorders, and conditions have associated communication and/or swallowing difficulties. Examples include an individual who might be status post cerebrovascular accident with aphasia and word retrieval or comprehension difficulties or an individual status post removal of vocal cord nodules to be evaluated for vocal hyperfunction and possible therapy. The following is an example of how such a referral might be stated:

> Robert Smith, a 78-year-old, was referred for a speech and language evaluation and therapy by his neurologist, Thomas Wolf, MD. It was reported that Mr. Smith experienced a cerebrovascular accident on July 12, 2022, and currently presents with aphasia characterized by word-retrieval difficulties and unclear speech.

Basic information concerning the referral is clearly provided and the purpose of the requested assessment is straightforward. Many times, especially in medically based referrals, a provided diagnosis accompanying the referral infers that subsequent therapy will most likely be needed. It may be assumed by the referral source that following the evaluation, the individual being assessed will then be enrolled in some type of intervention as determined by the evaluator. This type of referral process usually occurs when the clinician has established a successful relationship with a physician such as an otolaryngologist or neurologist and sees many of their patients.

The occurrence of comorbid medical conditions and communication disorders is not limited to adults. Children and adolescents also experience a variety of conditions with comorbid communication disorders. This can include a 3-year-old child following surgical repair of cleft palate needing evaluation and therapy or a 2-year-old recently diagnosed with cerebral palsy. Common referral sources to speech-language pathologists also include pediatricians, psychologists, and a variety of professionals from educational settings where a definitive co-occurring diagnosis may not be as clear. In these cases, the assessment of a communication disorder and resulting diagnosis could become the initial part of an eventual interprofessional evaluation that will lead to a diagnosis. Autism spectrum disorder, social pragmatic language disorders, learning disabilities, and childhood apraxia of speech are conditions that may be less clear initially and become more apparent with a speech and language evaluation as part of a broader interprofessional assessment. In those cases, a more general referral statement might appear as follows:

> Emily Johnson is a 3-year-old referred by her pediatrician, Jane Smith, MD, to rule out possible difficulties in the acquisition of speech and language.

An alternative statement might include a client who is being referred to "determine current level of communication." These examples should provide basic guidelines and not become routine boilerplate templates.

Referrals from educational settings, from preschool through secondary school, may also be targeted in their nature and come with specific examples of problems related to be considered in the assessment. Teachers, school psychologists, social workers, and parents may note school-related difficulties related to aspects of communication following observations, discussions between professional staff, or review of student work. Some of these reasons are noted in Table 4-1 for preschool and younger grades. These reported referral observations, educational concerns, and behaviors will

TABLE 4-1
Common Reasons for Referrals for Evaluation From Educational Settings

- Difficulty being understood by peers or teacher
- Not socializing with classmates
- Having difficulty in "circle time" with listening and/or talking
- Difficulty explaining, telling stories, relating events
- Grammar is awkward
- Difficulty remembering stories read in class
- Not using enough language with peers
- Does not follow directions, understand, comprehend
- Repeating sounds or words
- Specific language-related academic/literacy difficulties
- Difficulty with phonological awareness
- Difficulty organizing thoughts, expressing ideas
- Difficulty finding words

understandably vary by the age of the individual student. Description of areas of concern accompanying the referral helps in establishing an understanding of the reason(s) for the evaluation. They help in planning the assessment and should be noted in the statement that specifies the reason for referral. There can be countless reasons for such an evaluation, but whatever they are, they should be stated and documented as part of the written evaluation.

As children progress through school, reasons for speech and language assessments will often parallel curriculum demands. Referral reasons and descriptions of difficulty may include early and later elements of literacy, such as not remembering letters, problems with phonological awareness, and language problems associated with reading, writing, and mathematics. Difficulty with "word problems" is a common referral for a language evaluation as children transition into this integrated math and language level of mathematics learning. Social pragmatic difficulty with language may present throughout school years with the ever-increasing and changing demands.

Suffice it to say, the list of reasons for referrals is extensive. The inclusion of these reasons is an important part of each and every evaluation. Referring back to a report months or even years following the completion of the evaluation, the documentation of the reasons an evaluation was performed is an important and sometimes critical factor. To have it correctly and properly documented is important. The source of this information is equally as important.

THE INFORMANT IS IMPORTANT

It is important in providing a case history that the reader not only realizes the source of the referral but who the informant(s) providing the case history information is. Information that the evaluator will be documenting in a case history should be attributed directly to a source, and it should be clear what the source of a piece of information was should any question or discrepancy later arrive.

The provider of the information for the case history is described as the informant. The reader or eventual end user of the report should be clearly aware of where the information in the case history came from. This should also be clearly stated in the initial section of the report. It can be noted initially in the reason for referral or stated initially at the beginning of the case history. This can be easily and simply done and provides a clear reference to the reader of who served as informant. If an individual is an adult who comes alone to an evaluation and provides the relevant case history, the following can be stated initially in the report:

Mr. Smith was seen for a voice evaluation and served as an informant providing the following case history.

If the patient or client is accompanied to the evaluation by another individual, such as a friend or family member, who provides information, that should be noted as well. The following example is noted.

Mr. Robert Smith was referred for a speech and language assessment by his neurologist, David Johnson, MD, following a recent diagnosis of Alzheimer's disease. Mr. Smith was accompanied to the evaluation by his daughter, Jane Leston, who served as informant for her father.

Information contained in a case history should always be attributed to a source. The information may be obtained in a variety of ways. Many times, a patient, client, or family members will be asked to complete and return a case history form with questions targeted to the age and presenting problem(s) related to the individual being evaluated. This can be the patient or client themselves, family member, or someone familiar enough with the patient to complete the form. There is always a space to indicate the name of the person completing the form and their relationship to the individual being evaluated. It is currently more common for the case history form to be available online along with other necessary forms, such as insurance information, Health Insurance Portability and Accountability Act (HIPAA) forms, and information concerning procedures for the evaluation. It allows the evaluator to review all information prior to meeting with the client or patient and determine areas where additional follow-up questions may be required. Another possibility is for the evaluator to meet directly with the client or patient and informants to conduct the interview in person where case history information is collected. An advantage to this technique is that it allows the evaluator to establish initial rapport, ask more in-depth and follow-up questions as needed, and begin to actually assess the client or patient through the interview process. The disadvantage, of course, is the additional time required. It may require an additional session when evaluating children who the evaluator may not want present during the parent interview. The method will vary by setting, type of evaluation, personal style, and preference of the evaluator and time limitations. It is important that any way information is collected one must clearly attribute the source.

Information contained in the case history does not just originate directly from the client, patient, or family. Other sources of information are available, frequently used, and often required. When completing evaluations for students within school settings, for example, a Committee on Special Education will require information from multiple sources. This could include teachers, other therapists working with the student, or tutors working with the student at home. Information will be included in the case history section and must be relevant, clearly stated, and properly attributed to the source.

An evaluator may be asked by the individual being evaluated to review previous medical reports, evaluations from other professionals, progress reports, report cards, or any number of other documents that will contain information that will be important to consider in evaluating the communication abilities of a client or patient. An evaluator will also frequently request similar types of documents from a client or patient if they are available. The clinician may consider information contained in these types of documents relevant or significant enough to want to include the information in the case history. In such a case, the information should be properly quoted with specific reference as to the date, title of document, and the name of the provider. It should also be clear to the reader of the evaluation whether the information is directly quoted or is an evaluator's summary of information contained in the document. The evaluator, deciding on the level of detail they are comfortable with, can also state whether the documents were provided or obtained from the patient or client or obtained directly from the originator of the document. The following is an example of the manner in which the results of a student's recent neuropsychological evaluation might appear in a case history:

> As part of the current evaluation, a number of documents were provided to the evaluator by the student's mother (name) for review. A private neuropsychological evaluation dated January 22, 2022, by William Smith, PhD, included a diagnosis of "language disorder." Difficulties with language were noted throughout the report and indicated that "language deficits interfered in a number of areas including comprehension of questions, formulating answers, and reasoning skills."

CASE HISTORY

The case history section in a speech and language evaluation report is typically written in narrative form. Depending upon the requirements of a specific work setting, it can also be presented as a checklist or in a short-answer format as part of a questionnaire. Whatever the manner of presentation required, it is important to understand and be able to generate a basic narrative form that is typically taught and used in most graduate programs. The case history is presented at the beginning of the report, following the reason for referral, and orients the reader to relevant information necessary to understand the background information for the individual being assessed and the factors that may be important contributing elements to the eventual diagnosis. While the format of the case history varies from setting to setting and evaluation to evaluation, this is the next important segment of each speech and language evaluation.

Currently, many institutions are switching to or are currently using electronic medical records (EMRs) or case history form templates. These types of documents will present a preprogrammed listing of specified and important case history areas and questions required by the institution. The individual being assessed or the evaluator will complete the case history form presenting information in a brief, succinct, and easy format. With current advances in technology and the increased use of EMRs, these modifications in documentation make sense, save time, reduce paperwork, and allow for the clear transfer of information.

At this time, emerging professionals are exposed to EMR technology and documentation but continue to be trained in the more standard technique of producing a professionally written speech and language evaluation document in narrative form. Learning to produce a professionally written narrative case history enables the evaluator to understand the process of transferring information that was obtained from a client's case history form provided prior to an evaluation or the information obtained during an actual interview into a cohesive, logical, written format. Written evaluation reports are still required in many and varied settings. They continue to be used in most educational settings. The information contained in the case history may be relevant to third-party payers, reviewers who approve intervention and placement services, and in a variety of other required professional correspondence where specific results of an evaluation are required. Speech-language pathologists, therefore, must be able to accurately and successfully place required information in a written format and not just "check the box." The written process trains the speech-language pathologist to see the case history information cohesively, in a logical order, with salient information often becoming more apparent. This might not occur as readily or as easily from reviewing a list of preprogrammed questions. The preparation of the narrative format allows for review and understanding of the information contained. Writing a standard case history report further enhances and provides additional practice in professional written communication skills, which is an essential skill for all clinicians.

Professional report writing involves a specific style, phrasing, vocabulary, organization, and technique that requires learning, practice, and experience. It is a necessary and important part of professional training programs, and students often struggle with this aspect of their training. For those unfamiliar with professional speech and language report formats, it is quite different from the writing students and emerging professionals are accustomed to.

To begin with, providing information via an evaluation report is done in a less elaborated, more specific, objective, less personal, and more focused manner than traditional narratives usually are. Linguistic form is greatly reduced when compared to traditional narrative writing. The evaluator in writing a case history section must determine the important and relevant information to be included. The evaluator must become knowledgeable as to what is relevant and important by considering the statement of the possible problems, age of the individual being assessed, reason for the referral, and possible contributing diagnostic symptoms. Thus, for a 3-year-old who presents with a possible speech or language delay or disorder of unknown etiology, there is one set of case history information that will prove more relevant. A difficult pregnancy, complicated delivery, family medical history, or delayed developmental milestones may prove to be relevant or significant contributing information. This information is less relevant for a 45-year-old professional voice user being evaluated for vocal hyper-function or a 35-year-old with traumatic brain injury following a motor vehicle accident. Different sets of case history information will prove important with respect to the uniqueness of the reason for an individual's referral. In conceptually considering the written diagnostic report, a case history section is presented in each report. This remains a consistent part of the process in that a case history must be included with the evaluation and one can learn to write a case history. The depth and breadth of knowledge as to the questions to ask and necessary information to be collected will vary with the possible etiology of the speech or language disorder. The questions for an adult with fluency disorder are different from those for the parent of a young child with a language delay. The ability to recognize and determine these questions is a different skill set acquired through training and experience. The underlying concept of providing a "case history" and the reasons and necessity of doing so remain constant.

Once the desired information to be included is determined and collected, the actual organization of the narrative is determined. This will depend on the content of the information to be included. For a younger individual, a chronological organization may make the most sense and prove most efficient. This could include an order beginning with information related to pregnancy, birth, delivery, and developmental milestones. This could be followed by medical, family, school, and social history. For an adult with a communication disorder of neurological origin, beginning with the medical history followed by the individual's occupation, education, family, and social circumstance would make more sense. The individual and their presenting problem and reason for referral will ultimately determine the organization and information to be included. The next step will be to decide on the specific areas and how to best organize the information.

The amount of information collected for a case history can be extensive, and when the report is finally written, a determination will have to be made as to what to include in the final report. Since final reports are generally completed following the completion of the entire evaluation, the clinician will have had the opportunity to spend additional time with the individual being evaluated, learn to understand the patient better, gain additional ideas concerning the communication disorder or etiology, and have an opportunity to speak with other interested parties, including family members or referral sources. This process will eventually help in determining which information will be relevant to include in the final case history. The relevancy of the information to be included can become clearer as the evaluation progresses, and it is important to keep notes as to what specific information should eventually be included in the case history.

Report writing is a process, and presenting the written case history is just part of the process. It should be straightforward and does not have to be made more complicated than it is. The goal is to determine how best to simply present the necessary case history information. Consider it a necessary element of the report with a goal of providing background information. Recognize that this goal is different, separate, and apart from discussing the importance and relevance of the information contained in the case history that will later be used to help in the final synthesis of findings. The contribution, analysis, and understanding of the background information to final diagnosis will occur in the final sections of the report.

Table 4-2	
Examples of Case History Background Information	
CHILD	**ADULT**
• Prenatal	• Occupation
• Birth	• Work responsibilities
• Neonatal	• Medical history
• Motor development/milestones	• Medications
• Speech/language development	• Education level
• Medical history	• Hobbies/interests
• Family history	• Social
• Previous relevant evaluations	• Previous interventions
• Education	• Family constellation
• Play/social	• Current living situation
• Eating/feeding	• Allergy/diet restriction
• Current/previous interventions	• Hearing
• Hearing	• Languages spoken
• Languages spoken	• Family history
• Family constellation	• Emotional
• Caregivers' concerns	• Communication needs/concerns

The relevance of all of the information that is collected in a thorough case history and connecting relevance to diagnostic significance is an impossible task to present within this chapter. This goal would clearly require an entire textbook or more in addition to the academic coursework and clinical contexts necessary to understand the knowledge. Table 4-2 provides a list of some of the elements that need to be considered in a case history. These areas are familiar to most speech-language pathologists and are taught early on in academic training. The table is placed as part of review and reminder that the evaluator must decide which elements are necessary and relevant to include, as well as their meaning, as they become part of the analysis in the final assessment and diagnosis. The table breaks case history areas into those that are generally targeted toward child and adult assessments. Under each area suggested are broad categories with the realization that under each area are numerous related topics that may need to be explored. For example, under education and school-related areas, a clinician might inquire about specific difficult subject areas, relationships with teachers, progress, reading, writing, or ability to independently complete homework. General areas more appropriate for an adult case history are also suggested with the similar idea of there being numerous related areas that can be probed. An additional concept to consider is that the areas suggested do not consider the countless questions that will be presented specifically related to the reason for referral and problem. For a voice evaluation, the individual would be questioned specifically about vocal function, variability of voice throughout the day, or fluctuations in various parameters of voice, such as intensity or quality. Similarly, a fluency evaluation would entail additional questions targeted to stuttering such as difficult sounds or words and history and types of previous therapies. It is not the intent of this chapter to pursue all of the disorders and the questions that could be asked. This is covered in numerous courses, clinical experiences, and actual practice. That is not the "how" of the evaluation process, but the "how" of case history report writing. Once it is determined which elements of the specific case history are to be included in the report, it is the "how" of the report writing process that determines the best way to organize and present the information. One must present the information in a logical order and seek to combine significant relative and related areas succinctly, as well as state the information in a direct manner.

Organizing the Information

Once it is determined which information is to be included, it must then be decided how to best present it. Considering how much content there is in each area, the importance of each area, and the purpose of the evaluation, the evaluator can decide which content areas can be completed together and if subheadings can be used. If irrelevant, tangential, or unimportant information is to be deleted, eliminated, or reduced, that must also be decided.

The organization and presentation of this section, as are all sections of the report, is important for clarity and content. Should the evaluator wish to reference information contained in the case history in their summary and impressions or use specific relevant information in helping to support or determine a diagnosis, the information should be presented in a format that is easy for the reader to access. Case history information can be important in knowing what was, and was not, previously done to assist in making recommendations and referrals. The content and style of presentation of the case history rests in the hands of the evaluator.

The clinician must make the final decision as they are the only one with the entire picture of the patient or client when it is time to sit down and write.

A Subheading on Subheadings

In reading thousands of reports through the years, the author can state that the use of subheadings is one of the most variable stylistic decisions that occurs. Most clinicians will separate major sections, generally accepted within diagnostic report writing into such areas as reason for the referral or statement of the problem, case history or just history, behavior or observations, articulation, phonology or speech sound production, language, impressions, and recommendations. Even within these areas, evaluators sometimes choose to further organize the information into further subheadings within these sections. For example, this might include stimulability and diadochokinesis under a subheading of speech sound production or receptive, expressive, and pragmatic under a broader subheading of language. Since there is no one recommended and standard way to organize our reports, the variations in the way subheadings are used vary greatly from evaluator to evaluator and report to report. The differences in the specific organizational style are also a result of differences in training programs, supervisors, and work settings. While using the broader subheadings as described are at least somewhat more consistent and understandable between reports, the use of subheadings within the case history section seems to have less consistency.

In preparing reports, it becomes the responsibility of the evaluator to use and incorporate subheadings within the document when and where needed. The bases of these decisions would be to facilitate understanding and determine the most efficient and correct way to make the reader aware of salient information in the client's or patient's history.

A basic question when selecting the appropriateness and necessity of placing a subheading must be predicated on understanding their use. Simply stated, a subheading should be used to help organize a document. A properly placed subheading will facilitate understanding for the reader by providing a short topic summary of the content to follow. The subheading will also help the clinician in organizing the information to be presented into related areas, similar concepts, and collaborative ideas. The writer can determine the content relationships, easily see information that may be irrelevant or tangential to content presented under subheadings, and determine where additional or new information may be placed. A clinician must also determine, based on the content to be presented, if subheadings are called for. It becomes the responsibility of the report writer to consider this information, which further may explain the varieties and inconsistencies in their use.

In the case of a child, the information may best be presented chronologically. An emphasis and more detail would then be placed on the specific areas that appear to be important to or have a direct impact on the reason for referral. An adult with a significant medical history, communication problem that affects work or social life, and previous evaluations would require the case history to be targeted to these areas. There may be little, if any, reason to discuss developmental milestones and elementary school history. These become the decisions that must be determined by each individual evaluator based on the case, amount and relevance of case history information, results of the evaluation, and how they all intersect.

In evaluating a child with a history of prenatal difficulties, significant delivery, and complicated neonatal course, it would make sense to combine them into a section with a subheading of "Pregnancy, Birth, Developmental Milestones." One might then continue with subheadings that could include such areas as "Medical, Feeding, Hearing" and/or "School, Social, Play, Family." Should these aspects of the history and others be generally unremarkable and within age expectations, it could make sense to not use subheadings and present the information in a few paragraphs, in a more straightforward manner. A limited sentence such as "Pregnancy, birth, and developmental history were all uneventful as reported" would suffice to indicate all of these areas were unremarkable. A statement such as "Speech, language, and motor milestones occurred within age expectations as reported" would be enough to indicate to the reader that none of these areas were delayed. These statements are clear and provide the necessary information without excessive detail and elaboration. Even if something important or significant exists in the history, it can be presented in a concise manner, eliminating the need for a subheading. An example might be "medical history is significant for one febrile seizure at 12 months with a fever of 105 and an associated emergency room visit. Follow-up by a pediatric neurologist indicated no sequela and routine follow-up as needed."

In summary, the reason for referral and case history set the stage for the report that will follow. It orients the reader to what the evaluation is "all about." Conceptually, then, whatever the age of the individual, possible diagnosis, or severity, the report will begin in a similar manner. The only thing that changes is the reason the client is seeking assessment and the nature of specific questions to be asked and relevant responses. Thus, an evaluator will use a similar framework for initial documentation within each report based on their acquired knowledge and skills. The dilemma of deciding "how I should begin this evaluation" is avoided.

Behavioral Observation
That Is All You Need to Do

Communication occurs through modalities other than just verbal interactions. It involves a great deal more than just speaking and listening. Facial expressions, posture, gesture, a nod, a smile, or a tilt of the head all convey and enhance intended meaning. There are also nonspoken behaviors associated with the communication process that can interfere with communication. These are behaviors that interfere with the "back and forth" of communication, and some of these same behaviors can interfere with the clinician's ability to assess speech and language. It becomes the task of the speech-language pathologist conducting an evaluation to determine what underlying behaviors exist as noted during the assessment or outside observations that will result in the failure of the client or patient to comprehend, respond, or attend during an assessment. The behaviors observed during assessment may likely interfere with the communication act in more natural and daily contexts.

Specific behaviors or patterns of behavior may co-occur along with and can be indicative of underlying disorders. The underlying disorder or pathology in and of itself will cause disturbances in communication. The behavioral concomitant may exacerbate the already existing communication disorder. It is important during the speech and language evaluation to identify and note any relevant and significant interfering behaviors and, as importantly, document them in the final written diagnostic evaluation. Behavioral concomitants to communication difficulty may also be included in the initial referral request, and as such, it is important to look for these behaviors during the assessment.

Blaustein, S. H. *Diagnostic Report Writing in Speech–Language Pathology: A Guide to Effective Communication* (pp. 31-38).

They should either be included or ruled out as contributing factors in the diagnosis. The behaviors described and included in a final diagnostic report must be relevant to the assessment and diagnostic process, add contributing diagnostic importance, and be included as part of any summary and impression describing the patient's communication status. Such behaviors can be of such communicative importance that they will play an eventual critical role in recommendations and other interprofessional referrals for further assessment or intervention strategies to manage specific behaviors that interfere with the communication process.

Thinking About Normal

The speech-language pathologist, accepting the role of a qualified evaluator, uses any number of standardized tests, authentic measurements, informed clinical opinion, and experience to assess the many and varied aspects of a client's communication abilities. That is what we do. At the core of this process is the ability to determine expected performance on a task compared to what a patient or client is, or is not, doing. In explaining the process of assessment, notice the use of the term "expected" vs. "normal." In diagnostic report writing, the terminology used is important, and there can be subtle differences between words chosen. The vocabulary in a report should therefore be carefully selected. The eventual semantic content of a report can make a difference in a reader's overall perception of the elements contained within the report or the diagnosis itself. One word frequently used in speech-language pathology diagnostic reports is "normal." This concept, especially in reporting behavior, warrants some careful reflection. The reader is reminded of the necessity to carefully consider one's own understanding and awareness of cultural diversity in determining "normal."

The act of putting what one sees and judges into words requires such skill that adages such as "a picture is worth a thousand words" or "beauty is in the eye of the beholder" have come to describe the generally accepted idea that what we observe is dependent upon our own individual experience and judgment set. A primary difficulty in describing behavior is transferring what we see into a written format that will accurately reflect the clinicians observations. It is one of the report writer's challenges. This difficulty is not isolated to describing behaviors but oral structure, functions, gestures, play, and other elements of the evaluation that require subjective analysis and description.

If one were asked for a synonym or definition of "normal," words like typical, usual, common, standard, ordinary, or conforming appear. Further consideration of the topic may reveal that the concept of "normal" can vary specifically with respect to behavior. Normal behavior varies with time, setting, age, and an activity. One's behavior watching a football game in a stadium is quite different from one's behavior watching a ballet in a theater. In addition, culture impacts behavior, with each culture having learned expectations. This includes how one interacts and respects elders, how one behaves with those in positions of authority, interactions with professionals, or interactions with individuals of a different gender. Rules of eye gaze, proximity between speaker and listener, and even touch exist. The expectations and roles for children participating and interacting with adults vary with respect to learning, attention, and initiation of language. If an evaluator is accepting the role of completing an evaluation and assessing an individual's communication ability, which includes associated behaviors, then that evaluator is responsible for understanding all of these variables. In observing, documenting in one's notes, interpreting, and eventually reporting on behaviors, it is essential that the clinician is careful to understand the accepted differences in behaviors between groups. Understanding diversity should be an uncompromised and essential requirement for speech-language pathologists assessing behavior and, in fact, every aspect of the communication act.

Issues of recognizing diversity, not only in our assessments but also in our interactions with clients, students, supervision, and in our daily lives, have recently taken a spotlighted role and, rightfully so, are an important factor in our society. Aspects of diversity, including gender identification, race, culture, diet, and religion, must all be clearly understood when describing "normal." Normal, if used at all, must be described in terms of the variability of environmental expectation and the very acceptable variations in behavior that occur within diverse groups. Normal then becomes a term to use with caution and care. Psychologists, in determining normal from abnormal behavior, use psychometric test batteries, rating scales, interviews, and projectives and have specialized training in determining behavioral "norms." The *Diagnostic and Statistical Manual of Mental Disorders, Fifth Edition* (DSM-5; American Psychiatric Association, 2013) is used by psychiatrists, psychologists, social workers, and numerous other professionals, including speech-language pathologists, to determine diagnoses, lists behaviors that are necessary to determine and subsequently document when classifying and diagnosing patients. The behaviors described are often reported to be "consistent with" a specific diagnosis. Speech-language pathologists, in describing behaviors and their diagnostic significance, often rely on limited behavioral observations that have been conducted during an assessment conducted during a limited time frame and within a restricted environment or setting such as an office. In some instances, reports from parents or other informed sources are used to describe behavior and are included in reports without the assessing clinician ever seeing the behavior reported. This should be made clear. The limits in how "normal" is assessed must be considered in light of the assessment methods we use to arrive at conclusions.

Where and how the term "normal" is used with respect to behavior in a particular client or patient should be used following analysis, consideration, and thought. After all, what is "normal" attention or "normal" focus? What does "normal" relatedness look like? How much deviation does there have to be from whatever is considered "normal" for the assessment to be made that the displayed behavior is "abnormal"? These decisions are usually limited to subjective determination made exclusively by the speech-language pathologist who eventually will be accountable for these decisions and might very well be asked on what they are based. There must be a clear and accountable answer to that question. Proper documentation in one's notes and especially in the final diagnostic written report where this information is used and contained can assist in providing an answer to such a question whether it occurs months or years later. This may not be an unusual occurrence, as impartial hearings, reviews, later assessments, and reevaluations all require the evaluator to look back on what was done and said. This is contained in the evaluator's final diagnostic report. It should be realized that the use of the term "normal" extends well beyond behaviors observed. Reports often describe a "normal" tongue, "normal" pregnancy, or "normal" onset of first words. Normal is also frequently used in reports to describe a "normal" rate of speech or "normal" parameters of voice, including resonance and intensity. In describing behaviors (or elements of speech and voice), there should be clear underlying accepted and evidence-based information, if available, for the use of the term. A full description of what is being assessed and under which conditions it is being assessed will help. The use of a broader terminology such as "within normal limits" or "within age expectations" sets the picture of there not being one specific "normal" but an acceptable range within which adequate behaviors, performance of task, or visualization of a structure being viewed may fall. That is why we often read of tasks being done without difficulty, adequately, or successfully rather than a specific "normal." Many times in a case history, events are described as being "unremarkable." It might be stated that "birth history was unremarkable." The use of such terms suggests successful, without complication, or not out of the ordinary. This would imply that there is not one "normal" path that was not followed. Finally, the evaluator should be aware that when behaviors or elements of communication are not normal, typical, or adequate, by inference they are then abnormal, atypical, or inadequate. The possible subjective negative connotations that such terms may lead to, especially in the area of behavior, should be weighed on the impact of the eventual reader of the report.

TELEPRACTICE

Some basic considerations can create a framework that will enable clinicians to document their behavioral observations in a final report. To begin with, describe the setting. Observations are usually done during assessment sessions that occur in the clinician's office, but observations can also occur bedside in a hospital room, classroom, playground, or home. It is important for the reader's reference to indicate where the observation occurred. Pragmatically, behaviors are understood in terms of settings and therefore must be understood in context.

It is important to mention telepractice here where, as a result of COVID-19, the need to re-motely provide speech and language therapy to avoid in-person contact has dramatically increased. Clinicians must be aware of this platform if they are to provide distanced therapy as well as to appreci-ate and fully understand reports and documents where telepractice has been utilized. The American Speech-Language-Hearing Association (ASHA) has a dedicated section on its website and states, "In 2005, ASHA determined that telepractice is an appropriate model of service delivery for audiologists and speech-language pathologists" (ASHA, n.d.). ASHA, on its Professional Practice Portal, provides information related to client selection, environmental considerations, reimbursement, ethics, and other areas of which evaluators should be aware. The following guidelines from the Portal are pro-vided as they pertain more directly to evaluation and documentation through telepractice:

Clinicians should maintain appropriate documentation, including informed consent for use of telepractice and documentation of the telepractice encounter.

Clinicians should be knowledgeable about and compliant with existing rules and regula-tions regarding telepractice, including security and privacy protections, reimbursement for services, and licensure, liability, and malpractice concerns.

Clinicians who deliver telepractice services must possess specialized knowledge and skills in selecting assessments and interventions that are appropriate to the technology and that take into consideration client and disorder variables. Assessment and therapy procedures and materials may need to be modified or adapted to accommodate the lack of physical contact with the client. These modifications should be reflected in the interpretation and documentation of the service.

Many advantages of remote service delivery have become evident, and telepractice is becoming a routine part of modes of service delivery. As such, it is important to become aware of telepractice regulations and guidelines, and the reader is advised to become knowledgeable in this area.

The use of telepractice creates a new lens with which to view client and patient behavior for evaluators to be aware of. Differences in assessment, test selection, test administration, and docu-mentation need to be addressed. Certainly, settings that occur in person are different from remote practice. The evaluator and client or patient not being in the same room but viewing each other on a computer monitor requires a different set of behaviors and observations. Furthermore, the fact that these encounters may take place on laptop computers, iPads, or even cell phones requires new interpretations for attention, reciprocity, and consistency of response, eye gaze, and relatedness. It must also be noted that most standardized assessments are based on statistical analyses and psy-chometric determinations that are centered on responses that have been collected "in person." It is therefore necessary to specify the nature of the interaction, and a comment is required stating that the assessment instruments have not been standardized for the platform in which the test is being administered. We are seeing greater availability of standardizations for tests where data on remote administration have been gathered, but this is the exception rather than the rule. One should also be aware that if an in-person assessment is conducted, the use of masks and face shields should be indicated as well. The lack of opportunity to visualize the examiner's mouth or for the examiner to visualize a patient's or client's mouth does, to some extent, limit information that is acquired via facial expression and lip reading. Any difference in test administration that varies from the instruc-tions in the examiner's manual should be specified, and a client's or patient's behavior should also be specified with respect to the setting. This should clearly be understood by the reader. If an evaluation is completed via telepractice, a statement should be provided in the evaluation indicating the remote nature and possible implications. The following is such an example.

Note: Due to COVID-19, this evaluation was conducted remotely. All testing was com-pleted using a HIPAA-compliant Zoom platform. The tests that were administered during the assessment are not standardized or norm referenced for remote administration. Scores cannot be reported but test performance will be described. Tests and subtests were carefully selected to include tasks that would be least affected by a remote administration and not re-quire aspects of in-person assessment, such as directly sharing materials, objects, pictures, or test items. Pictured stimuli, as needed, were presented digitally or presented using a Hue camera. Behavioral observations will also vary as lack of in-person contact may impact attention, eye gaze, reciprocity, consistency of response, engagement, and other aspects of interaction that may be better demonstrated during face-to-face contact.

Behaviors not only vary by setting but also by activity, which clearly plays a key role in an individual's responses. Speech-language pathologists have assumed an increasing role in diagnosing and providing interventions for social pragmatic language disorders and pragmatics in general. Activity and context is critical in pragmatic assessments but also plays an important role in the assessment of behaviors that may occur in any communication disorder. What is occurring during the interaction where behaviors are described must be explained to fully understand the associated behaviors. Activities are an important factor in determining unexpected, atypical, or inconsistent behaviors and, as with setting, the activity being conducted must be understood in describing a client's response.

A specific behavior in a specific sitting during a specific activity best allows the reader to understand the impact and degree of the activity on the response. Informal assessments, the use of play with toys, games, sustained listening to repetitive questions or prompts during a task, writing or reading, and authentic response during discourse are all examples of activities where the communication demands will vary and, as such, a patient's responses will vary.

Another observation that should be documented is what, if anything, elicits a specific behavior. While behaviors can be self-initiated, spontaneous, or random, they are usually associated with some preceding event. From the point of view of behavior analysis, behaviors can be viewed as a response to a specific stimulus, or perhaps a set of stimuli, that "triggers" a response. The antecedent behavior may be seen as linked to a resultant response, and response can be judged as appropriate or inappropriate, acceptable or unacceptable, typical or atypical, or within a range of normal (as previously discussed). Behavior, therefore, can be viewed in an additional context of what "causes" the behavior. The determination of this cause can be a very important part of the evaluation and a contributing factor in determining the eventual diagnosis and, as importantly, enabling the evaluator to decide on necessary therapeutic and intervention strategies. Whether self-initiated and spontaneous or linked to a specific prompt, demand, or task, behaviors that interfere with the assessment process or communication must be described. The impact of any of these behaviors should be considered and included in any summary and impression provided if significant.

Not all behaviors that warrant description and documentation in the final diagnostic report are necessarily spontaneous, random, or in response to an identified stimulus. Behaviors may exist as part of an underlying diagnosis and are just comorbid realities to the individual having such a diagnosis. For example, a patient who presents post cerebrovascular accident who has a right hemiparesis that affects gait and ability to hold a writing instrument in their dominant hand presents with an observation that must be made as an impact on written communication. Similarly, lability, exaggerated emotional reactions, also associated with cerebrovascular accident, is an example of another comorbid behavior that should be noted, as it should be understood as it is related to the communication act and may become a variable in therapies and interventions. There are similar behaviors that occur with traumatic brain injury, dementia, or a variety of neuropathologies, that are comorbid with the diagnosis, affect aspects of assessment and communication, and therefore should be noted.

Once the clinician determines that an observed behavior is present and in some way is relevant to the assessment, diagnosis, or possibly eventually the intervention process, the frequency and duration of these behaviors should also be considered. This can be an indicator of the level of the behavior's possible impact on communication and will help in determining an overall degree or measurement of the severity of interference a behavior may cause. This would be an additional useful measure to present in the report if it can be determined within an evaluator's degree of confidence.

Asking for a repetition of a prompt, question, or comment is not an unusual behavior. Such requests following most utterances or questions produced by the evaluator warrant noting. Similarly, younger children may exhibit a brief tantrum associated with frustration or fatigue during an assessment. This is to be expected. Excessive tantruming during an assessment with difficulty regulating a return to baseline level of behavior or causing the evaluation to terminate prematurely as a result of this behavior might be noted if it occurs on repeated attempts at examination. Not only can description of these types of behaviors explain results of the evaluation, but they will also aid in eventual summary, impressions, and recommendations as significantly interfering behaviors may result in additional interprofessional assessments to further assess, document, and determine the severity and presence of such demonstrated behaviors.

SOME DESCRIPTIONS ARE MORE DIFFICULT THAN OTHERS

One of the most difficult aspects of documenting behavior is the description of an actual behavior. In describing behaviors, an evaluator must be careful not to overinterpret, mislabel, mislead, diagnose, or be judgmental. It should be a behavioral observation, and as such, in this section of the report, it should be an objective description of the behavior observed by the examiner considering the elements previously described. The meaning of behaviors observed; their implication, inference, or relevance to the final diagnosis; recommendations; and referrals will occur in the final summary and impressions section. The observations of behaviors during an assessment will be analyzed and interpreted within the parameters of the context and woven into the final evaluator's conclusions as part of the total results of the assessment. Salient, significant, and consistent behaviors will be logically integrated into the evaluation. Properly documented, they will be seen as valuable confirmation that provides additional support for writing one's conclusions, recommendations, and additional referral for interprofessional assessments or interventions if needed.

The aspects to be included in a behavioral observation described thus far are more easily observed, charted, and recorded for analysis and description and therefore more straightforward to describe. They are more objective by their nature. The actual behaviors that clients and patients exhibit can be more abstract and less objective, and their determinations and meanings must often be inferred. They are more qualitative in nature and difficult to quantify.

These behaviors and the terms that describe them are studied, explained, and observed in clinical training and should be familiar to clinicians before they begin their Clinical Fellowship. One's ability to accurately describe, understand, and see all of their manifestations, expressions, and influences on communication continues as long as a clinician continues to evaluate and provide interventions for clients and patients. This can be a lifetime of clinical practice. For these reasons, the objective of this discussion is not to explain the behaviors to be described in an evaluation but to provide an overview of how to present them in a clinical report.

These behaviors include joint attention, distractibility, opposition, and relatedness to name a few examples. Attention is an area that is frequently described in reports. Yet to fully understand attention is to realize that there are numerous forms of attention, including sustained, divided, and alternating. Table 5-1 presents a list of possible behaviors to be observed that are typically covered in diagnostic courses and should be familiar to most graduate students. One must understand what these look like, the communication demands they support, and how to accurately convey to a reader where possible deficits lie. Their impact on an individual's receptive, expressive, or pragmatic language and how they relate to a diagnosis must be discussed in the diagnostic report.

What behaviors to document is a very difficult question for the evaluator. "What" actual behaviors to include and their relevance is part of a clinician's training and experience and, again, is not the purpose of the present discussion. What needs to be considered for objective diagnostic report writing is "how" to document behaviors in question. The "what" is learned through numerous courses completed in graduate study, completion of one's Clinical Fellowship, and perhaps through years of clinical practice. An entire text could certainly be devoted to specific significant behaviors, or sets of behavior, that should be noted and described in reports as being relevant and associated with a plethora of disorders, diseases, or traumas that are comorbid with communication disorders.

TABLE 5-1
Examples of Areas to Consider for Behavioral Observations

• Aggression	• Localization
• Attention—auditory	• Neglect
• Attention—sustained	• Opposition
• Attention—visual	• Physical concomitants
• Distractibility	• Play
• Imitation	• Relatedness
• Impulsivity	• Responsiveness
• Initiation	• Reticence
• Intentionality	• Social engagement
• Joint attention	• Tracking
• Lability	

TABLE 5-2
Factors to Consider in Reporting Behavioral Observations

- Describe the setting during which behavior occurs.
- Describe activity during which behavior occurs.
- Describe any specific antecedent behaviors, if present.
- Describe frequency and duration of behaviors observed.
- Objectively describe the behavior to be reported.
- Do not diagnose behaviors observed.

Consider that executive function, a critical area of study for speech-language pathologists, is the term that incorporates planning, inhibition, attention, and memory. Executive function is involved in both activities of language and behavior. The comorbidity of attentional issues, emotional issues with language issues, has been well documented to be quite high. Neuropathologies, neurosurgery, dementia, and stroke all may lead to symptoms that affect both behavior and language. Many of these disorders are progressive in nature, with language function and behavior functions diminishing over time, unfortunately. The understanding of these interrelationships is critical to speech-language pathologists conducting assessments of individuals across the life span. Understanding the concept that these behaviors need to be observed if present, well documented, and cohesively and correctly integrated to provide the results of assessment and diagnosis is critical. Absent this information, if present and relevant, the resulting report will be incomplete. Table 5-2 presents a summary of factors to consider when documenting behavioral evaluations in a diagnostic report.

REFERENCES

American Psychiatric Association. (2013). *Diagnostic and statistical manual of mental disorders* (5th ed.).

American Speech-Language-Hearing Association. (n.d.). *Professional practice portal-telepractice.* www.asha.org/Practice-Portal/professional-issues/telepractice/#collapse-1

Speech Sound Production
Writing Clearly About Clearly Speaking

Disruptions in speech sound production are a concomitant of many communication disorders, and, as a result, their assessment and accurate documentation is an important component of many, if not most, speech and language evaluations. A thorough description of findings explaining speech sound production, detailed analysis of productions, impressions, and, when determined, an accurate final diagnosis must appear in the written final evaluation report. Difficulty with speech sound production is a symptom of or result of numerous disorders and conditions. Difficulty with accurate speech sound production may reduce overall intelligibility to varying degrees in the speech of toddlers, children, adolescents, and adults. Conditions such as cleft palate, cerebral palsy, childhood apraxia of speech (CAS), phonological process disorders, and articulation disorders are familiar to clinicians who work with children. Adult-associated disorders that impact production of speech sounds include stroke and Parkinson's disease to name but a few examples of etiologies that will impact speech production throughout the life span. The structure and function of the oral peripheral articulators may be compromised following surgery for malignancies or damaged as a result of trauma such as a motor vehicle accident affecting the ability to produce the speech sounds necessary for articulate speech. It even falls within the scope of practice of speech-language pathologists to analyze the speech sound production of individuals with accents and regional dialects who wish to modify their production for a variety of reasons. The causes of reduced speech intelligibility are varied and broad in scope. The nature and degree

Blaustein, S. H. *Diagnostic Report Writing in Speech–Language Pathology: A Guide to Effective Communication* (pp. 39–50).

of difficulty of the impact on speech production will result in levels of severity that can range from an individual who is mildly difficult to understand to someone who may be completely unintelligible to the listener.

The speech-language pathologist assessing speech sound production must not only have confidence and the depth and breadth of knowledge to competently assess speech sound production, but also possess the ability to transfer that knowledge into a well-documented report that a reader can conceptualize, understand, and imagine what the evaluator has heard. It is a task not to be underestimated in difficulty. Radiologists view X-rays, CAT scans, and MRIs and describe and interpret what they see. The actual visual images can be sent along with written reports to further enhance understanding for the reader. The speech-language pathologist must analyze and interpret an acoustic signal into graphic written description and interpretation. There is no other concrete information to rely on other than the description provided in the report that readers hold in their hands. The description of speech sound production must therefore be clearly and accurately presented. The evaluator must have the skill to correctly, clearly, and succinctly document what they are hearing, analyzing, and interpreting into written form.

The proper evaluation of speech sound production is an important and necessary component of speech evaluations. Without a precise, clear description and analysis of the standardized and authentic techniques and measures used, specific presentation of results, and diagnosis with necessary recommendations, this aspect of the speech and language evaluation will be reduced in effectiveness. It will have reduced value to the client and the necessary eventual intervention planning. It is incumbent on the evaluator to not only complete a thorough, competent evidence-based evaluation using appropriate assessment measures and techniques but to then be able to competently present the results in written form. The results will be needed for a variety of reasons, including determining etiology, planning intervention, establishing baseline function, or making appropriate referrals for additional assessments.

The purpose of this chapter, as in other chapters of this book, is not to provide instruction on how to assess speech sound production. We proceed on the assumption that the reader has the basic knowledge and skills to evaluate and analyze this aspect of communication but is then faced with the task of how to most efficiently, accurately, and effectively transfer this information to the reader via the written diagnostic evaluation. There are numerous textbooks, courses, and online resources available that can assist in the "how" of the actual speech sound production assessment process for those who require review.

WRITING ABOUT SOUNDS

There are many aspects of assessing speech sound production that can make this a difficult construct to put on paper. As with other aspects of communication to be assessed and documented in the speech and language written report, there are no standard, required criteria as to what to include, how to organize the section, and how to report findings. This will be done based on the training, experience, and work setting. These will vary from training program to training program, setting to setting, and evaluator to evaluator. The first question might actually be what to title this particular section of the report. Reporting the evaluation of speech sounds within a report will generally have its own section with a subheading.

According to the American Speech-Language-Hearing Association (ASHA) Practice Portal, (n.d.) a speech sound disorder is "an umbrella term referring to any combination of difficulties with perception, motor production, and/or the phonological representation of speech sounds that impact speech intelligibility." This broad definition under the term "speech sound" covers a wide spectrum of etiologies that may include aspects of motor production and perceptual and phonological disorders. Reference to anomalies and deficits in structure or development of any of the articulators is absent from the description. The Portal then goes on to list a possible classification schema that includes speech delay, speech errors, and motor speech disorders that include dysarthria, apraxia of speech, and motor speech disorders not otherwise specified. Given the lack of a unified and widely accepted speech sound disorder classification system, what most obviously needs to be assessed and presented in a systematic and comprehensive manner is the client or patient's ability to produce speech sounds and an inventory of those sounds.

Sound production is the foundation of intelligible speech and consists of an individual's repertoire of consonants, vowels, and the ability to combine them into units of varying length and complexity. The successful ability to produce and sequence sounds, at its most elemental level, allows transfer of oral language. An assessment of speech sounds will result in findings of adequate production or possible disruptions in speech sound production that may, based on analysis of assessment results, be attributed to any number of possible etiologies or conditions that hopefully will be further specified in the report. An appropriate title or subheading for this section might then be Speech Sound Production, although headings of Articulation, Phonology or Articulation and Phonology are often used. This author, given that articulation disorders and phonological disorders are distinct etiologies unto themselves, prefers the broader heading of Speech Sound Production to describe the information to be included in this section of the report. This heading would seem to be clear and simply suggest to readers across disciplines that it is an individual's speech sounds that are being evaluated. When included in a speech and language evaluation report, it is recommended to have at least some heading for this section that will clearly differentiate speech sound production from elements of language for the reader. Any subheading for a report's content area must be clear. It is surprising how many individuals who are not speech-language pathologists do not understand the difference in the terms, speech, and language, as they are used by our profession.

The problem then becomes how an evaluator reports an individual's speech sound production given the wide variety of possible etiologies, numbers of possible types of errors to be described involving a quantifiable number of individual speech sounds, and an exponentially greater number of possible combinations of speech sounds, a multitude of possible standardized test choices, informal assessment techniques, and ever-changing environmental contexts and demands. This does not include the various theoretical bases of how best to assess speech sound production with new information introduced from journal to journal. It almost seems easier to do the assessment than to actually write about it. Realizing the complex components involved, the clinician must systematically incorporate each piece into a document that must be presented to the reader that will result in a clear presentation of an individual's speech sound production ability. With practice and experience, it will allow for the evaluator to develop a mental template for documentation and eventually make for easier, more efficient diagnostic report writing. Conceptualizing a basic process for documentation of assessing speech sound production will allow for generalizing the documentation process across patients and clients. Remember that although etiologies, patients, and ages may differ, the basic assessment requirements remain similar and a process for presenting the results can follow a similar process. With that in mind, a clinician can be less apprehensive about approaching a disorder not previously encountered as each disorder does not necessarily demand its own strange or novel testing. It is true that specific tests may exist for certain disorders such as apraxia or dysarthria, but the concept that a standardized speech test should be used is the construct to be understood.

At Least One Standardized Test Is a Good Place to Start

An assessment of speech sounds typically begins with the selection and administration of a standardized test. Remember that standardized tests may or may not be norm referenced so consideration should be given to the specific test selected. Most of the available standardized speech sound assessments are familiar to clinicians and allow for systematic assessment of sounds based on the underlying theoretical model of the test selected. Most are norm referenced, include a variety of ways to assess speech sounds, and provide a scoring system and specified way to analyze results. These features provide a straightforward way to begin the evaluation of speech sounds and, as importantly, provide the examiner with a generally accepted way to assess and analyze the results. This will facilitate documentation of the results in the written report. This is another extremely important area where the evaluator must be aware of multilingual and multicultural aspects of speech sound production. Careful attention must be paid to the use of standardized norm-referenced testing.

Begin by specifying and describing any norm-referenced or criterion-referenced standardized tests that were included in the assessment. It is assumed that the specific chosen test will have been selected based on the age of the individual, the reason for referral, and relevant case history information. The assessment measure should target eliciting and assessing speech sounds in an evidence-based manner considering the patient or client, reason for referral, and the evaluator's best hypothesis as to a possible etiology. The evaluator's theoretical beliefs underlying models of speech sound production should be taken into consideration and hopefully align with the test(s) selected. Initially selecting the most appropriate test measure will not only be important to the actual evaluation, but eventually an appropriately chosen test will facilitate documentation and reporting. While some professionals may recognize and be familiar with the more common tests of speech sound production such as the Goldman Fristoe Test of Articulation-3 (Goldman & Fristoe, 2015), which was first published in 1969 and remains in large use today with its third edition published in 2015, there are many other valid, reliable tests that are also available. Many of these tests have also been updated, provide specific and useful assessment information about speech sound production, and provide for a variety of quantitative and qualitative measures that will enable and facilitate a way to report results. The speech sound production section will then begin with the full name of the test administered, including the number of the most recent edition used. Using "Goldman Articulation Test" as a title is not sufficient if one actually used the third edition and the correct complete title of the test is not provided.

They are not the same test. In fact, while readers may understand the test being referenced, no such test exists. It can be misleading and perhaps unethical. Abbreviations should not be used the first time a test is mentioned but may follow the initial statement of the name of the test in parentheses if they are to be used later in the document.

Many times, the title of the test is sufficient to give the reader a basic idea of what the test assesses. It is clear that the Arizona Articulation and Phonology Scale-4 (Arizona-4; Fudala & Stegall, 2017) assesses articulation and phonology. The number 4 following the title indicates the test is in its fourth publication, which means, there are likely to be updated norms, revisions, and possible changes in content or analysis to reflect previous critiques, current trends, expanded uses, or other changes that will keep an assessment instrument current. This is the case for most tests where the name is followed by a number. Evaluators should always use the most current version of a test. The Frenchay Dysarthria Assessment—Second Edition (Enderby & Palmer, 2008) is a test for dysarthria, and the Kaufman Speech Praxis Test for Children (Kaufman, 1995) is a norm-referenced test for apraxia. Providing the full name of the test is good documentation and report writing practice, and the actual name of the test in and of itself can be descriptive and informative.

Once the test is named, it is usual to state the reason it was used. It might be stated that "The _____ Test was used to assess targeted speech sounds in single word productions." The purpose of the test may also be stated or summarized as provided by the test authors in the examiner's manual. For example, "The _____ Test was administered. According to test developers, this test provides an evidence-based way to assess the articulation skills of children ages 3 to 6 in single-word contexts." Further description of the test may include stating the manner in which speech sounds are elicited. A statement such as "The _____Test requires the ability to name pictures of common objects as presented by the examiner to the examinee with targeted sound(s) embedded in the label for each picture presented." Once this is stated, the reader will understand what was done to elicit the sample of speech sounds to be assessed in a standardized manner. This straightforward introductory statement will clarify the nature of the standardized testing for the reader.

WRITING WHAT WE HEAR

One of the biggest challenges in documenting the speech sound production section is determining how to present the actual speech sounds as they were produced during the assessment to the reader. This determination involves including in the report the sounds that were correctly produced and the sounds that were produced in error. There are a number of decisions to be made if one is to approach this process in a logical manner. The first decision is to determine which speech sounds produced by a client or patient should be documented in the evaluation report. Is there a need to document the speech sounds that were produced correctly by the individual being evaluated? The answer would usually be no. Standardized assessments contain numerous targeted sounds that are elicited in a variety of ways. Scoring is generally on the number of targeted sounds produced incorrectly. There are various ways to convert the number of error sounds to comparative qualitative and norm-referenced metrics. The point is that the focus of assessment is on the sound production errors. That is core to the reason for referral, and the focus of assessment should be on the determination of the type, frequency, and nature of the error sounds produced. That is what should be documented with the idea that sounds not identified as produced incorrectly are produced correctly. We know what correct productions sound like. An exception would be if the evaluator is attaching a fully completed response protocol answer sheet from the articulation test administered to the report or is producing a chart or grid that lists all required responses made by a client. In that case, all targeted sounds would be presented, but the focus would continue to be on sound production errors. It should also be realized that some standardized test scores may include percentages of incorrect productions to be used in intelligibility or other ratings, so at least, some understanding of the nature and number of all sounds targets could prove helpful. It may not be necessary though to include all of the correctly produced sounds. In the context of an actual report, it is generally not necessary to list all of the vowels, consonants, consonant clusters, vocalic /r/ environments, and other sounds that are correctly produced. It would prove too lengthy and is unnecessary. An exception would include a sound that was previously produced in error that at the time of the evaluation through development or intervention is currently produced correctly. This would typically be reported by an informant.

It is next necessary to document the actual speech sound errors that do exist. Initially, these would be the error productions of targeted sounds as determined by the specific administration requirements of any standardized tests used. Evaluators should be aware that these sounds are not universal to all speech production tests. The nature of the speech sound production test selected and the specific targeted sounds contained in the test stimuli and the nature of how they are conceptualized will determine the error sounds to be indicated in the report. As the targeted sounds and errors produced will also serve to determine test scores and resulting interpretations, it further illustrates the need for the evaluator to carefully select and correctly administer the speech sound production test to be used. The selected test will determine the error sounds to be reported. These are the sounds that will also contribute to the level of reduced intelligibility and will aid in determining the severity of the disorder. They will be analyzed along with other information gathered on speech sound production to determine possible etiology or diagnosis. Note that as standardized as this appears, it remains the responsibility of the evaluator to listen to the sound productions and determine their accuracy. This will be based on each listener's judgment of acoustic accuracy.

The individual error sounds reported will initially be determined by the speech sound production test selected. The evaluator must then report the results as specified within the test examiner's manual. This is a very straightforward process. The manner in which the sounds are reported will be determined by the nature of the test and the theoretical manner in which the test developers have selected specific sounds and incorporated them into stimuli, typically pictures to be named by the examinee. These are designed to elicit the speech sounds in a prescribed manner. The reporting of the results will then be the specific speech sounds of each individual test and will vary by each test eventually selected by the evaluator. Although the sounds are understandably the sounds of the English language, their frequency of occurrence and position within words will vary depending upon the constructs of the developer and the way it is theorized that speech sounds should be evaluated. Some tests incorporate vowels while others do not. In some tests, sounds are weighted as to their frequency of occurrence in the language. Other variations exist. English-language speech production tests are assumed for this discussion, but it should be realized that articulation tests are available in languages other than English. The evaluator must also determine if sound production testing in second languages should be administered.

There Are Different Ways to Assess Sound Productions

Speech sound production tests may evaluate sound productions conceptualized as articulation errors or phonological processes. There are many tests available that assess both articulation and phonological processes in the same assessment instrument. This is often indicated in the name of the test where both manners of analysis are included. The benefit of such a test is that the same elicited stimuli can be used to assess articulation and the phonological processes that occur. In some instances, a few additional stimulus items are added to complete the necessary phonological process analysis. Articulation tests are also available that "pair" with a different phonological process assessment, which again are efficient in that they utilize the same stimulus items for both assessments. Many of these assessments are available with computer-assisted scoring that make analysis of the responses easier for the clinician to compute. In summary, the basis and source of the individual referral, case history collected, and the examiner's ultimate test selection will drive the initial set of speech sounds to be assessed, including the manner in which they will be assessed. The evaluator's responsibility is then to accurately and clearly transfer the information, collected in a standardized format, to the evaluation report. The qualitative and quantitative information collected under the speech sound production section will be used and analyzed. The evaluator's additional use of the data, interpretation, relevant comments, and findings will then be used in the summary and impressions to assist in arriving at a possible diagnosis.

Reporting Standard Speech Production Results

Each standardized assessment of speech sound production will provide a way to determine raw scores from responses. Various conversion tables will also be provided by test authors to allow the evaluator to derive meaning from the raw scores. The raw score usually is determined by the total number of speech sound errors or phonological processes noted during the client or patient's productions. This can occur at a word level, sentence level, or both. These raw score error "summaries," once converted, will break down the articulation or phonological process errors into a variety of qualitative and quantitative areas. Many are standardized, and comparisons to age-matched peers can be determined. As previously discussed, there are no universally accepted terms to describe the interpretation of each individual test's raw scores into qualitative interpretations. The use of diagnostic terms such as articulation disorder or phonological disorder is generally understood, at least by speech-language pathologists. Other diagnostic interpretations are less clear, vary from test to test, and are based on each individual speech sound production test's conceptual underpinning and developers' determination of how results may best be analyzed and presented. Many tests enable the use of a descriptive severity level. This, when included, is determined by test score results, including number of errors. When using severity levels, it is important to note how severity was determined based on the test interpretation and that the level was not subjectively determined by the evaluator. Table 6-1 presents examples of some of the types of information that can be determined and reported from just a few widely used articulation and phonological assessments currently available. A review of the table provides examples of the ways speech sound errors are interpreted on different tests. The report should contain the analytical diagnostic terms contained in each standardized test used along

TABLE 6-1

Standardized Speech Production Reporting Terminology Examples

GOLDMAN FRISTOE TEST OF ARTICULATION-3

- Overall intelligibility rating
- Intelligibility percentage
- Stimulability
- Sounds-in-words vowel error analysis
- Sounds-in-words phonetic error analysis
- Sounds-in-sentences phonetic error analysis
- Sounds-in-words R error analysis
- Standard scores, percentile rank

KHAN-LEWIS PHONOLOGICAL ANALYSIS-3

Core Phonological Process Summary

- Number of occurrences
- Percentage of occurrences

Supplemental Phonological Process Summary

- Number of occurrences
- Percentage of occurrences
- Processes per word
- Vowel inventory

ARIZONA ARTICULATION AND PHONOLOGY SCALE-4

Articulation

- Word articulation total score
- Sentence articulation total score
- Speech intelligibility interpretation value
- Word sentence articulation critical difference score
- Level of articulatory impairment
- Percentage of speech improvement for retesting

Phonology

- Level of phonological impairment
- Severity range of phonological error patterns
- Percentage of occurrence
- Standard scores, percentile scores

with test scores. The meaning of each diagnostic area must also be explained for the reader to fully understand how speech sound production is being interpreted. Even experienced speech-language pathologists may not understand categories for reporting some of the data if they are not familiar with the nature of the test that was used.

Completing and documenting the test results of the speech sound assessment used based on the constructs provided is important but will not provide the reader with the specific speech sounds errors produced. This will require a direct transcription of the error sounds to be documented in some way along with the correct target sound and specific stimulus. The nature of articulation and phonological process assessments is to use the quantity of sound errors produced to determine one's overall performance ability. Standardized tests do allow for further analysis of types of errors, but these are usually interpreted using supplementary tables and descriptors and may not be used for determining basic scores. The limitations and advantages of speech sound production tests should be recognized by the skilled evaluator to properly use scores effectively in reporting results and interpreting those results.

It is necessary to document the actual errors produced during the standardized assessment based on the construct of the stimuli to be tested. For example, in an articulation test, if the target test sound is /k/ in the word "bike" (elicited from a picture), a child may produce the word "bite." According to the examiner's manual, this could be considered a /t/ for /k/ substitution in a "final" word position. This may also count as one point toward a final "raw" error score. If the test were assessing phonological processes, this could be viewed quite differently. The same error would be considered "fronting" and count as one point toward a number of total phonological processes occurring throughout the test and a score of one for the specific "fronting" phonological process. The reader must be made aware of these differences, which can only be done through careful and proper documentation and explanation. It must be realized that the differences between the manner in which the identical error is viewed will be most evident to a speech-language pathologist. Other professionals who must somehow make use of the report may not fully appreciate the differences involved. Accurate and clear report writing is therefore essential.

Since there is no recognized, standardized way to present these individual speech sound errors in a written report, the determination of how to document and present sound production errors must be made by the evaluator. However it is done, it must be remembered that the documentation must be complete, accurate, and presented in a way that is organized and makes clear to the reader which targeted speech sounds are incorrectly produced. It is also important to remember that when writing the speech production section, it is not necessary to provide an etiology or cause at this level of the report. Analysis of errors such as "developmentally appropriate" and/or errors that are a result of "unilateral lingual paralysis" can be provided in a summary and impression session. Speech errors are initially being presented as "data" that will be analyzed along with additional information that will be elicited numerously during the assessment. The oral peripheral examination, to be discussed later, will be of particular importance in evaluating speech sound production.

The evaluator is again faced with questions of documentation. Should errors be transcribed using the International Phonetic Alphabet (IPA) or in some other way? It is a question that requires some thought. Speech-language pathologists are trained to use IPA transcription, which provides a more specific detailed description of speech sounds and will allow for more specific and detailed transcription of errors. Speech-language pathologists are trained in the use of the IPA in graduate school and transcriptions are practiced. Phonetic transcriptions should be recognized and understood by speech-language pathologists. It is how and what we are trained in. It is a tool of our trade, and it is the most effective and straightforward way to indicate speech sound productions. One must consider that in deciding to use IPA transcription, there are some drawbacks. Most individuals beyond speech pathologists will not be familiar with the underlying sounds many of these symbols represent. The inclusion of the IPA transcription will be most useful to other speech-language pathologists who would perhaps be accepting the individual being assessed into an intervention program. The second consideration is that many speech-language pathologists, unless using IPA regularly, may not remember the IPA or be familiar with some of the less frequently used symbols that represent many of the error sounds or atypical errors.

(articulation sound errors are noted below:)

Target	Sound	Correct	Actual	Error Type
DOOR	r	/dɔr/	/dɔ/	Omission /r/
HAMMER	r	/hæməˑ/	/hæmə/	Omission /r/
SHOE	/ʃ/	/ʃU/	/tu/	Substitution t / ʃ
SLIDE	/d/	/slaɪd/	/slaɪ/	Omission /d/
TIGER	/r/	/taɪgəˑ/	/taɪgə/	Omission /r/
THUMB	/θ/	/θʌm/	/tʌm/	Substitution t / θ
VACUUM	/v/	/vækum/	/bækjum/	Substitution b / v
FROG	/fr/	/frɔg/	/fɔg/	Omission /r/

(phonological errors are noted below:)

Target	Sound	Correct	Actual	Process
SHOE	/ʃ/	/ʃU/	/tu/	Stopping
THUMB	/θ/	/θʌm/	/tʌm/	Stopping
SLIDE	/d/	/slaɪd/	/slaɪg/	Backing

Figure 6-1. Reporting articulation and phonological errors.

In making this seemingly simple decision of whether or not to use phonetic transcription, one might consider that a speech-language pathologist will eventually be the one most likely to use the report functionally. It makes sense to specifically, efficiently, and effectively transfer the most appropriate information to the professional who will actually be functionally using it. The second consideration is that if speech-language pathologists are accepting the responsibility for assessing speech sound production and documenting results, it is appropriate to recognize the responsibility of learning, using, and being functionally able to use an effective tool of our profession. Professionals in other fields do not restrict their reports to lay terminology or simplify critical data. It becomes the responsibility of the reader to infer the meaning or, if necessary, use readily available sources to understand the meaning. The speech pathologist can assist in making the report more understandable by using the phonetic transcription and if necessary use more straightforward orthographic representations. If the client or patient produced a /th/ for an /s/ substitution during a test (think/sink), the writer may use th/s to illustrate the substitution. Figure 6-1 presents an example of how speech sound errors may be presented in a report using IPA transcription. Note that examples are provided for listing both articulation and phonological errors. There may be a need at times to list both types of errors within a report as children may often present with both types of errors. This reinforces the idea that the evaluator must be knowledgeable and careful in their choice of tests and that both types of specific errors must be reported.

In summary, when reporting speech sound errors, it becomes necessary to not only quantify them, convert them to scores, and use qualitative descriptors specifying severity according to individual test guidelines but to also effectively provide a specific listing or inventory of each error. This is a critical component of the final report. This will allow readers to understand the nature of the speech sound errors, provide a clear baseline of errors at a point in time (date of report), and, if needed, enable a starting point for initiating a plan of intervention.

REPORTING AUTHENTIC SPEECH SOUND PRODUCTION RESULTS

As with all components of a communication evaluation, the evaluator must rely on a variety of techniques to assess speech sound production. Measures not only include administering a variety of standardized tests, but the use of authentic "informal" assessment must also take place. These measures, subjectively based, will provide the reader with the evaluator's "informed clinical opinion" as to the nature, severity, and characteristics of any possible speech sound disorder. Standardized and authentic assessments both have advantages and disadvantages that evaluators should be aware of. The standardized, decontextualized, specific nature of speech sound testing relies on words being produced at the single word level, short phrases produced in a context that usually elicit responses via pictures. A client or patient's speech sound productions, for a variety of reasons, may not mirror speech produced during natural, spontaneous conversation. There are a number of reasons for this, not to be explained here, but include the fact that the shorter utterances and the client or patient's awareness that their speech sound production or intelligibility is being measured may cause them to produce speech more slowly or clearly then in the natural context. It is therefore necessary for the evaluator to include in the diagnostic evaluation an assessment of speech produced in a more natural context. Samples may be elicited during play, conversation, or, in some instances, asking a family member to provide a recording of the patient's speech during a variety of natural activities that the client or patient typically engages in.

The evaluator, following standardized testing, will have a baseline of a client's speech sound inventory based on the standardized testing and can then measure the individual's spontaneous productions against the decontextualized inventory. The components for the documentation of these assessments are similar to those previously described in documenting most standardized assessments.

The context and manner of the authentic speech sample elicitation, tasks involved in collecting the sample, and duration of the sample should be specified to allow the reader to understand where and how the speech sample was collected. If speech was sampled in a variety of contexts and environments, they should be specified as well. Any differences in the authentic speech samples across these contexts should be pointed out and explained. Possible contextual factors influencing differences in spontaneous productions, if determined, should also be explained.

An initial statement of overall speech intelligibility should be provided. It must be specified that unlike a severity determination that is based on specified criteria in a formal test, the severity level determined by the examiner is subjective and is based on the examiner's opinion and personal assessment. This will be based on experience and individual clinical judgment. This may be stated as "overall intelligibility of spontaneous speech was subjectively judged to be perceived as fair based on the examiner's clinical judgment." Note that terms such as poor, good, or excellent may be used depending on the sample. It may also be possible to use terms such as "fair to good" or "good to excellent" if the levels are not solidly within one range or vary between ranges. The examiner may also state that "unintelligible segments" may have been noted or that there were factors that impacted on speech intelligibility. For example, a rapid rate of speech in a client or patient with only mild speech sound production errors may present with further reduced intelligibility as a result of the rapid rate. Increased rate of speech may place greater demands on motor planning, resulting in less precise production of speech sounds. These factors should be specified and detailed in the evaluation report. This is the type of information revealed in authentic contexts. Reduced speech intelligibility is not solely the result of disordered speech sound production. Reduced intensity, resonance, and disordered vocal characteristics such as hoarseness can also serve to reduce overall speech intelligibility. These factors are not part of standardized speech sound assessment but clearly serve to reduce intelligibility. They can be critical diagnostic factors that are revealed during authentic assessment and further illustrate the importance of the informal context. They must be reported and described in the written evaluation, and their inclusion will have diagnostic significance and lead to more appropriate intervention planning and referrals.

The examiner should also provide and document specific examples of sound production errors that occurred during spontaneous, authentic conversation. It is very possible that the errors occurring during spontaneous speech closely resemble the errors that were noted during standardized testing. This should be stated and specific examples of spontaneous productions may be provided, illustrating the same errors that occurred during formal testing. It is also possible that types and numbers of speech sound errors may be greater during spontaneous speech, resulting in greater reduced intelligibility. The occurrence of articulation or phonological errors that were not noted during standardized tests often exists. It is important to note these as well and specify the additional speech sound errors that were clinically determined by the evaluator. In some cases, although less frequent, intelligibility and speech sound production may be better than that noted during standard assessment. Again, this should be noted.

Assessment of speech sound production is an important and critical aspect of any report. It is a difficult task to both complete and document speech sound production. When the evaluator has a conceptual understanding of the evaluation process and how to convert that process into a written format, it makes the documentation easier. It enables a better understanding of a client or patient's speech sound production and translates to a better written report, enabling greater understanding by the end users of the report.

STIMULABILITY

In documenting speech sound production results, the concept of stimulability is an important factor that must be included and falls within the speech sound production section of the report. "Stimulability" in speech sound production assessment refers to how "stimulable" the examinee is in being able to correctly produce the error sound(s) noted during the evaluation. The examiner uses modeling, explanation, and prompting to determine an individual's ability to improve their speech sound production. Stimulability is included on many standardized speech sound production tests, and specific directions are provided as to how to elicit the correct productions of the sounds found to be incorrect based on the test stimuli responses. This may occur at the sound, word, or sentence level. The significance of the stimulability task should be understood by the evaluator to be able to properly administer, assess, understand the implications, document, and incorporate findings into the final speech and language evaluation. A statement such as the following should be included:

John was stimulable to correctly produce the /s/, /z/, and /sh/ following modeling and instruction by the examiner. Stimulability for /r/ was poor. John was unable to correctly produce or approximate /r/ following modeling and prompting.

TWO DIAGNOSES TO HIGHLIGHT: APRAXIA AND DYSARTHRIA

Two specific diagnoses that can severely impact speech sound production, reduce overall intelligibility, and make the speaker's message difficult to understand include dysarthria and apraxia. These diagnoses, along with the case history and other determining factors, are largely based on the assessment of speech sound production. The diagnosis of dysarthria and apraxia occurs with sufficient frequency that they warrant highlighting in this section. Their assessment, analysis, and documentation of results follow a similar pattern to the procedures and processes for the articulation and phonological process disorders previously discussed. Remembering that evaluation and documentation follow a conceptual framework of basic procedures and documentation, one can address these specific disorders in a similar manner to that of assessing other disorders of speech sound production. Knowing the process facilitates the assessment and documentation, and the difference occurs because they are different disorders to be assessed.

Dysarthria is a neurologically based disorder affecting, among other areas, the oral peripheral speech musculature. The neurological impact is a deficit in the rapid, precise movements necessary to produce speech sounds accurately. The referral information for a patient with dysarthria will likely carry information related to the neurological condition that resulted in the dysarthria. The referral may also indicate a request to evaluate and treat a disturbance in speech following a specific neurological event. Adult neuropathy such as Parkinson's disease, amyotrophic lateral sclerosis, stroke, or traumatic brain injury may be suggested in the specific referral. For children, a diagnosis of cerebral palsy is often associated with dysarthria. The referral then will generally in the case of dysarthria suggest the etiology. The case history obtained by the evaluator will provide additional and necessary information. There may also be associated eating, swallowing, voice, rate, or intensity issues that may be reported and will need to be assessed and documented. Specific standardized tests for dysarthria are available and should be administered with results documented.

Apraxia in adults can also be a neurologically based condition that results in deficits in motor planning of speech sounds. Unlike dysarthria, articulation disorders, and phonological process disorders, where the errors are consistent and can be documented as a constant interruption of specific speech sounds, a hallmark characteristic of apraxia is inconsistent, randomly occurring errors. The oral peripheral articulators are not weakened. Oral apraxia may also exist, impacting nonspeech oral movements. The speech pathologist, based on referral and case history information, would suspect a possible apraxic component and then plan an appropriate assessment strategy. It must also be stated that apraxia is noted to occur in children with such incidence that a specific diagnostic term, childhood apraxia of speech, has emerged. Much attention has been given to this difficult-to-diagnose disorder, and information is readily available in journal articles, in continuing education programs, and on the ASHA website. Standardized tests are available for adult and CAS and should be administered and documented if apraxia is suspected. Sections of many tests for aphasia and other adult neurological disorders will also assess speech sound productions.

Diagnosing apraxia and dysarthria is emphasized in all graduate training programs with charts commonly used to illustrate differences and similarities. Analysis of speech sound production, along with case history and oral peripheral examination, are key areas to establish the diagnosis.

As with all areas in a speech and language evaluation report, accurately and appropriately documenting these three areas is critical.

REFERENCES

American Speech-Language-Hearing Association. (n.d.). Speech sound disorders articulation and phonology. https://www.asha.org/policy/pp2004-00191

Enderby, P., & Palmer, R. (2008). *Frenchay dysarthria assessment—Second edition (FDA-2)*. Pro-ed.

Fudula, J., & Stegall, S. (2017). *Arizona articulation and phonology scale—Fourth revision (Arizona-4)*. WPS.

Goldman, R., & Fristoe, M. (2015). *Goldman-Fristoe test of articulation 3* (3rd ed.). Pearson.

Kaufman, N. (1995). *Kaufman speech praxis test for children*. Wayne State University Press.

Khan, L., & Lewis, N. (2003). *Khan-Lewis phonological analysis (KLPA-2)*. Pro-Ed.

The Oral Peripheral Examination

A Mouthful of Description Will Suffice

STRUCTURE AND FUNCTION: DESCRIBING KEYS TO SPEECH PRODUCTION

Precise speech sound production is the result of a multitude of complex interrelated processes and functions that include respiratory effort, laryngeal coordination, resonance, and articulation. This does not include the remarkable contributions of neurological systems, including motor planning. At the core of this remarkable ability to produce intelligible words through sound production is the rapid, accurate, overlapping targeted movements of the lips, tongue, mandible, and velum acting within the intact structure of the oral, nasal, and pharyngeal cavities, allowing individuals to create the sounds of speech. This sensitive system, when functioning without defect, disruption, or disorder, enables humans around the world to produce the countless sounds and sound combinations that underlie the languages that are spoken throughout the world to enable civilizations to communicate.

In order to ensure that our clients and patients possess the intact ability to produce speech, the integrity of the necessary structures used to produce speech and unimpaired function of the speech motor systems must be evaluated. Any deficits in these areas must be ruled out as possible contributors to any reduced ability to produce speech sounds. Results of this critical assessment must

Blaustein, S. H. *Diagnostic Report Writing in Speech–Language Pathology: A Guide to Effective Communication* (pp. 51-59).
© 2023 Taylor & Francis Group.

TABLE 7-1
Common Reasons for Examining Oral Peripheral Structures

STRUCTURE	COMMON AREAS OF EXAMINATION
Face	Symmetry, dysmorphology, signs of syndromes, structural anomaly, hypo-/hypertonia, scarring
Dentition	Occlusion, arrangement, missing teeth, hygiene
Lips	Motility, range of motion, symmetry, strength, habitual posture, closure, bilabial compression
Tongue	Color, size, frenulum, range of motion, strength, carriage, motility, symmetry
Pharynx	Structural anomaly, tonsils, adenoids
Hard palate	Rugae, arch height, width, scarring, cleft, contour
Velum	Symmetry, motility, uvula (bifid), intactness, gag reflex, structure

be clearly documented. The oral peripheral examination is an essential part of speech and language assessments where there is any question of limitations in structure or function or any question of reduced intelligibility of speech. The evaluator must thoroughly assess both the structure and function of the oral peripheral articulators, which is what the speech-producing mechanism is commonly called. The ability to include this specific, targeted evaluation is core to the "speech half" of our profession of speech-language pathology. A disruption in structure or function as the result of illness, accident, trauma, congenital anomaly, or any other number of possible outcomes will impact the precise processes that produce intelligible speech. This disruption may be easily noted and significant or can be subtle and minor and still affect sound production. Sometimes something as simple as an individual having dental work such as a crown or bridge to replace central or lateral incisors changes the quality of sounds that clients notice and are troubled by.

According to the American Speech-Language-Hearing Association (2016), it is within our scope of practice to assess structure and functions of the oral peripheral articulators. The results of the oral examination assessment must be competently documented and presented in the final written diagnostic report. These results, depending on the findings, may prove integral to the final understanding of a speech problem and perhaps lead to, or be part of, an eventual diagnosis. In many cases, it is often tied to the initial reason for the referral and included in the statement of the problem as presented by the patient or referring source. This may include a patient with a neuropathy resulting in peripheral weakness or a surgical procedure causing structural change.

The importance of intact structure and function of the articulators is stressed in any number of graduate courses in speech pathology. Students may study the significant structural deficits that may occur in cleft lip and palate and the debilitating effects in function as a result of paralysis in amyotrophic lateral sclerosis. The associated speech and related communication difficulties in these disorders fall within the realm of the speech-language pathologist to assess. It is not necessary to provide a list of the structures and functions that are assessed in an oral peripheral examination as they are contained in basic textbooks and covered in all graduate programs. To stress how important this part of an evaluation is, however, Table 7-1 presents a list of oral peripheral structures that all impact speech sound production in one way or another and the areas that should be thoroughly assessed and documented. In keeping with the intent of this book, it is not the purpose of this chapter to provide the "how" to complete an oral peripheral examination but rather to suggest the "how" to objectively and accurately report the results of such an evaluation. There are numerous books, courses, and continuing education programs that are provided to teach the actual task of completing the oral peripheral examination. Less attention is given to the documentation of results.

WHAT TO INCLUDE

If we begin with the idea that physiological gestures of the articulators ultimately determine the acoustic end product (speech sounds), then it follows that any alteration in this gesturing (articulation) will produce a resulting and associated alteration in the planned target sound or sequence of sounds. Likewise, having an intact structure of the articulators and oropharyngeal cavity is critical to correct sound production. Any alteration in structure will result in changes to speech sound production. The evaluator must therefore rule out problems with structure and/or function of the speech-producing mechanism as a contributing etiology to disorders of speech. Documentation of the findings follows. The extent and degree of disruption affecting an individual's speech intelligibility will vary from mild, where a listener can perceive the speech message and it is generally understood, perhaps with a few missed words and phrases, to severe, where very little, if any, of the message will be understood.

Specifying and documenting the nature and extent of interference to speech sound production as a result of deficits in structure and function of the articulators is an essential component to the final written diagnostic report. It allows the reader to appreciate and understand what sounds are impacted, the effect of the impacted structure or impaired function on the ability to correctly and consistently produce speech sounds, the relationship between the disruptions and any more general etiology, and the degree of severity. The impact on overall speech intelligibility, stimulability, prognosis for improvement, and ability to compensate as a result of disordered structure and/or function must also be determined and documented. Thorough documentation of this section of the diagnostic report leads to recommendations that will include intervention strategies involving possible therapeutic, surgical, and/or prosthetic approaches. In the current professional climate where interprofessional practice is at the forefront of medical care, the need for additional interprofessional referrals for further evaluation and intervention becomes critical. Positive findings in any area of oral peripheral structure or function will necessitate appropriate referrals for additional evaluation or follow-up. Correctly documenting the oral peripheral examination is a significant section in the final evaluation report.

ORAL PERIPHERAL CONSIDERATIONS

Student training, coursework, and continuing education programs highlight the techniques, processes, and theoretical bases underlying the oral peripheral examination. Other common targeted educational experiences involve strategies to provide interventions based on the results of the oral peripheral examination. Far less attention is paid to how to correctly document these results in a written diagnostic report. There is little uniformity across settings and clinicians. Results are relegated to a checklist or a short paragraph or two without fully presenting an adequate description or understanding of the impact of oral peripheral articulator function or dysfunction. The results of this evaluation must also, if applicable, be included in the Summary and Impression section, which considers all of the results of the evaluation toward describing the patient's overall communication functioning.

As with all other disorders that speech-language pathologists treat, there are individual practitioners and specialty centers that perform oral peripheral evaluations in varied and more targeted ways that may be better than others. Such centers may have specialized instrumentation to measure or visualize structures and functions. They may be more comprehensive in their assessment and have individuals with specific experience and training for certain disorders, and the sheer volume of cases seen of a particular disorder and the related resources available should be considered as a possible referral option if one is uncomfortable performing this section of the evaluation. One such example would be speech disorders associated with cleft palate and craniofacial disorders.

It is important to also highlight that at least some of the cost for rehabilitation and interventions for individuals who have disorders associated with oral motor functional or structural deficits may be covered by third-party payers. Medical necessity is often a required factor in a report as a prerequisite to approval for coverage. Documentation needs to be very specific. It is important to identify and explain the structure and functional disruptions, the relationship of the deficit to any speech sound production or resonance disorder, and the relationship to any overlying etiology, disorder, or health condition. The prognosis for improvement should be included with specification for the needs and types of interventions. This must be clearly evident and understood by claims reviewers, which is an additional reason to carefully document this section of the report.

Thoughts on Documenting Oral Peripheral Function

With an understanding of the role of the oral peripheral examination, the practical problem then becomes how to document the results of this assessment. It would seem that this should be a rather straightforward task. In many ways, it is. The objective in writing becomes to clearly describe both the structure and defect, where applicable, and the function and deficit, also where applicable, of each of the contributing oral peripheral articulators. The challenge becomes that this can largely be a subjective evaluation. While there are some more objective ways available to describe various structural anomalies related to disorders, such as classification systems for cleft lip and palate, degree of ankyloglossia, or categorical systems for dental malocclusions, there are many other deficits that are harder to describe. Many are not part of any uniform classification system, and it becomes the responsibility of the evaluator to put what is seen into words. Congenital malformations, structural defects following surgery, and injuries following trauma or accident are but a few examples of events that may result in disruption of structure and function that will require precise description based on the evaluator's observations. The observed disruptions to the speech sound system will impact accurate productions and must be described following visual observation by the speech pathologist completing the examination. Accurate description, although subjective, must be done. A similar problem exists where the speech-language pathologist must report on the function of the articulators. While reportedly objective measures exist, such as diadochokinetic rates to describe rapid alternating speech sound productions, there have been questions in the literature as to their reliability and utility. Diadochokinesis will be described later in this chapter.

In the basic oral peripheral evaluation, the client or patient is asked to perform a generally accepted set or series of movements or gestures involving the lips, tongue, velum, and mandible. These procedures are learned during graduate training. Results of the examination are then qualified and quantified in a manner determined by the clinician to describe the success or limitations for each of the movements and structures observed. This is another area that many graduate students have limited experience with, and it is often practiced on classmates or individuals with unimpaired speech production systems. Students are lucky to be involved in training programs where there is opportunity to evaluate clients or patients with oral peripheral deficits related to a variety of etiologies.

In an actual examination, findings may include reduced movement of one or more articulators as the result of paresis (weakness) or paralysis (no movement), imprecise or compromised movements, structural congenital anomalies, or defects as a result of accident or surgery. Asymmetrical structure, asymmetrical function, and any number of other observed problems with accuracy, timing, and speed of movement may also be noted. Many of these observations will be understandably subjective based on the clinician's perspective and experience. For example, reports often attribute difficulties in speech sound production to hypotonia or muscle weakness. This is largely determined on visual inspection. A speech-language pathologist completes the oral peripheral examination and somehow determines that hypotonia is present. While there exists instrumentation to actually measure the strength of these articulators, these techniques are currently largely used in research settings and there is not readily available instrumentation that is regularly used in day-to-day clinical practice. Thus, terms like mild, moderate, or severe weakness or mildly impaired lingual lateralization are used based on the evaluator's knowledge, experience, and skills. Another common finding in reports of children with articulation disorders is a notation of "jaw sliding" or "mandibular instability." Lacking a clear clinical system for classifying and categorizing many of the variations in structure and function of the articulators that occur, the reader's understanding and interpretation are based on the impressions gleaned by the description provided by the clinician who performed the evaluation. This will largely be based on the evaluator's own frame of reference, techniques, skill, knowledge base, experience, or work setting.

Explaining by Writing

The procedures and techniques for completing an oral peripheral examination are usually well taught and practiced in simulations and actual supervised clinical practicums. They are basically understood by graduate students as they enter their Clinical Fellowship. What is less clear may be how to document the examination. The style, content, and organization will vary from program to program, setting to setting, and instructor to instructor. An understanding of the necessary components relating to the structure and function of the oral peripheral articulators as they impact speech sound production should logically lead to what aspects must be correctly documented. The final documentation of the oral peripheral examination should be complete, clear, succinct, and relevant. The documentation can be conceptualized into a number of questions that must be summarized and accurately described in this section of the report.

In evaluating structure, it is obvious that the structures being evaluated must be stated. Most oral peripheral examinations will include assessing the face, lips, dentition, mandible, hard palate, velum, and oral pharyngeal area. Structure must be correctly identified in the text of the diagnostic report. As the basic structure is noted, the area in question can be further specified. A more precise description of any defect indicating left, right, unilateral, bilateral, anterior, posterior, superior, inferior, upper, or lower will further clarify structural involvement. The size or extent of a defect will further clarify the description for the reader. In examining each structure, reporting on any significant findings and then clearly specifying not only the structure but the specific area and size or extent in question containing an anomaly, deviation, or defect will enhance documentation. For example, in the case of a patient who had a cyst removed from the tongue, the examination might indicate:

> A small postsurgical scar, characterized by discoloration and a slight raising of the area approximately 3 mm in length and 2 mm in width, is noted on the anterior central lingual segment extending posteriorly from the tongue tip.

Not only is the structure involved being described, but the reader will have a clear visualization of any defect of the structure in question. Once the structure is identified the function, if relevant to speech sound production, can be explained and documented. Each structure has an important anatomical and physiological function as it relates to speech sound production. These are the functions that the clinician has been trained to evaluate and consists of the tasks that the client or patient is asked to perform or imitate. Consider that all structures have function but only certain structures involve direct movement. The teeth, alveolar ridge, and hard palate serve important functions in speech production in resonance and in contact points for articulation. The maxillary segment of dentition and hard palate do not move independently without movement of the head. Lower dentition only moves in conjunction with the mandible. Disruptions in these immobile "functions" are related to structural defects that will impact acoustic output depending on their extent and severity. Their role, however, is passive in nature vs. other oral peripheral structures that are mobile and active, require motor planning, and have movements that must be initiated and actively demonstrated by the patient.

Labial function, for example, consists of retracting, pursing, and compressing the lips. Movements can be unilateral to the left or to the right and the lips can retract bilaterally. Lingual function may involve extension, retraction, elevation, depression, and tensing of the lingual muscle surrounding the outside of the tongue, resulting in "spooning" that occurs during sounds such as /sh/. Retroflexion may also occur. The velum elevates bilaterally and visualization of unilateral movement only can be indicative of potential difficulty. This is where theoretical knowledge comes into play, as the evaluator must recognize the typical structures and functions and realize what may be atypical to the degree that speech sound production will be altered. This must be documented in the final written report. Theoretical knowledge may further be employed where the evaluator must know that visualization alone of velar function is limited and a thorough assessment cannot be performed without objective visualization using techniques such as nasal endoscopy. Furthermore, in assessing the velum, structures such as the tonsils and adenoids may be involved in assisting velar pharyngeal closure, and their structure and presence may assist in or impede velar function. This information needs to be clearly specified for the reader and can have important diagnostic impact on eventual etiology, explanation of speech sound production, and the need for additional and more specialized evaluations or interventions.

After identifying the structures to be assessed and the necessary functions of these structures, one must indicate the client's or patient's ability or inability to execute the necessary functions as described. This is largely based on the evaluator's subjective description of how, or to what extent, the client or patient successfully completes the requested maneuver. Often, successful movement is described as "normal." It is difficult to use the term "normal" as there is much variability in function. "Normal" function can be on a scale of ability, which can result in adequate movement for sufficient speech sound production. Individuals can have disruption in function but have learned to compensate and will have successful end result speech sound productions. This can be described as well. For the purposes of evaluation, the use of a term such as "adequate" for speech production would provide a more appropriate description. The oral peripheral articulators, adequate for eating, chewing, or swallowing, should also be considered. Lingual elevation can be considered in relation to the necessary movements required to produce the lingual sounds, including lingual dental, lingual alveolar, or lingual velar. It is important to recognize that a client or patient may have some visualized restriction or mild weakness in movement that still allows for adequate speech sound production. This should be noted, as a sudden or gradual limited range of movement not previously present may be indicative of early-stage pathology and a baseline should be established toward monitoring patients over time. Appropriate referrals should also be documented.

It is more critical to document, note, and describe functions that restrict, limit, or impede movement and notably disrupt speech sound production. These may be inadequate, unsuccessful, imprecise, or poorly executed. The challenge becomes how to describe unsuccessful movements of articulators that occur rapidly in time in a way so that a reader can understand the type and degree of difficulty.

Consider that articulatory gestures or movements must be targeted to a desired point and move in a specific direction. This can be a starting point for describing accuracy of articulatory gestures. If a patient is asked to alternate touching the corners of their mouth with their tongue, it would require lateral tongue movement crossing the midline, perhaps starting right to left (direction), and the desired target would be both corners of the retracted lips. If contact were not made to either target on either side of the mouth, that would be a straightforward description.

> With lips retracted, the patient was able to lateralize the anterior lingual segment from the midline to the left labial corner, initiate movement toward the right corner, but unable pass the midline and make contact with the opposite side.

It might also be simply described as "the patient was unable to lateralize the tongue to the right past the midpoint of the lips."

Once the target and direction are described, it is necessary to describe the quality of the movement. The concept of "quality" is also very subjective, dependent upon the evaluator's visual interpretation and experience. Subjective descriptions of movements that are frequently used include awkward, effortful, poorly coordinated, or weak. These terms serve to give a greater picture of the patient's attempts to perform the desired voluntary oral motor gesture. As subjective as these terms can be, in the absence of pictures, drawings, or videos, the more description provided, the better the reader can understand the existing difficulties with oral motor movements. The previous example, if decided upon by the evaluator, might be expanded to include the following.

> With lips retracted, the patient was able to lateralize the anterior lingual segment from the midline to the left labial corner, initiate movement toward the right corner, but unable pass the midline and make contact with the opposite side. Subjectively, lingual movement was slow and the tongue appeared hypotonic.

Other factors may interfere with outcomes of desired movements of the articulators, and they should also be described. In the previous example, if associated difficulties with the lips or mandible were observed to further interfere with the task, they should also be reported. The patient might be unable to "disassociate" lingual function from other articulators, which would be an important fact to note in the diagnosis or intervention. A short lingual frenulum may restrict lingual elevation, retraction, or lateralization. The inability to stabilize the mandible or other structures while attempting to produce isolated voluntary movements may interfere with accuracy of movement of a targeted structure being assessed and the ability to successfully complete the movement required. Labial paresis or paralysis or associated labial movements that co-occur or interfere with lingual gestures should be noted. Tremors, fasciculations, and flaccidity are a few examples of described symptoms that are visually observed and subjectively described in reports. As imperfect as the system may be with a high reliance on subjective terminology, the greater the degree of specificity and clarity in the document, the better the reader will be able to understand the impact on the oral peripheral articulators as the result of possible underlying etiologies. Speech pathologists familiar with writing and reading reports will have an understanding of what these terms mean, however subjective, and the general understanding of many of these terms will provide added meaning to the reader who may be unfamiliar with oral peripheral exams. More specific description of areas of concern in the oral peripheral examination will allow for better explanation when the evaluator describes the relationship between deficits in oromotor function to speech sound production and overall intelligibility when documenting summary and impressions. The following is an example of what an oral peripheral examination summary for a child with an articulation disorder might look like in a diagnostic evaluation.

> An evaluation of the oral peripheral articulators was completed. Facial, labial, lingual, palatal, velar, and oropharyngeal structures were intact and adequate for speech production. Dental structure was significant for a Class III malocclusion (angle) and missing upper right central incisor. On imitating oral movements, labial and velar function were adequate. Difficulty was noted with lingual lateralization and protrusion as (name of child) was unable to disassociate the tongue from the mandible, and lateralization and protrusion of the mandible were observed as the tongue was noted to move in association with mandibular movement. Inability to elevate the tongue within the oral cavity was noted with associated head movements as the chin raised superiorly. Difficulty disassociating the tongue from the mandible was again observed on attempting lingual elevation.

Another common observation may occur when a patient or client will use an additional structure to assist in imitating a movement. This can also be indicative of difficulty with disassociation. Note the following description.

> When asked to elevate the tongue, the patient supported the anterior lingual segment with upper and lower lip compressed against the tongue and attempted to use the lower lip to elevate the tongue.

TABLE 7-2
Reasons to Clearly Document Oral Peripheral Examination Results
• Identify and understand causal relationships between structure, function, and speech sound production.
• Determine extent and severity of difficulty and determine appropriate intervention goals and barriers to speech intervention.
• Determine necessary interprofessional referrals, including for surgical correction, orthodontia, prosthetics, or neurological assessment.
• Specify impact of deficits in structure and/or function to third-party payers and reviewers for determination of reimbursement, qualification approvals.
• Clarify specific strengths and deficits to facilitate patient, client, and family counseling.

The extent of the oral peripheral examination may include additional maneuvers, techniques, and tasks that yield additional information regarding the structure and function of the articulators that will ultimately be responsible for accurate speech sound production. Many of these tasks are commonly performed but require integration of multiple aspects of oral motor functioning. If relevant, informative, and necessary, these tasks might include blowing, "puffing" cheeks with air, and sustaining this task while the examiner places pressure with their fingertips on the cheeks. Deficits may subjectively be demonstrated by the presence of nasal air emission or air "escaping through weakly sealed lips." Evaluators may also use a tongue depressor and ask the patient to lateralize, depress, or elevate the tongue against resistance provided by the examiner holding the blade against various areas of the tongue. This informal, subjective measure of "tongue strength" is another subjective, easily administered task.

Evaluators using such techniques as part of their oral peripheral examination must understand that these maneuvers are subjective, based on the evaluator's own opinion as to what the results mean, and the meaning of any difficulty with these tasks. They are not standardized, so one must be careful to clearly document exactly what was done, the difficulties noted, the results, and eventual interpretation of success or failure of the patient to complete these tasks. The possible diagnostic significance of failure to accomplish these tasks must be understood as they relate to deficits in anatomy and physiology, and their inclusion and use can have value diagnostically and in determining potential interprofessional referrals for more thorough and objective analysis. There are numerous reasons to complete and clearly document the results of an oral peripheral examination. Table 7-2 summarizes a number of these reasons.

DIADOCHOKINESIS

Diadochokinesis is a term that refers to the ability to rapidly sequence speech sounds. It is a measurement that is used to determine the rate at which a series of rapidly alternating sounds can be produced by an individual. Although it involves the production of actual sounds and unlike the oral peripheral examination that is primarily a visual observation, the diadochokinetic results are typically reported in the oral peripheral section of the final report. This would be appropriate as it is technically used as an additional measure of function in assessing rate of sound productions. Structure and underlying functional deficits can both reduce the accuracy of speech sound productions in attempting to rapidly sequence speech sounds.

The results of determining diadochokinetic rates are believed to be largely related to neurological function underlying articulation. It is believed that this measurement is useful in differentiating subtypes of dysarthria and other disorders, including traumatic brain injury. Detailed analysis of the nature of the sequencing difficulty and the manner and consistency of sound sequences produced may also be used in assessing apraxia of speech.

Despite the use of diadochokinesis for more than 60 years, questions remain as to how the task is specifically administered, interpretation of results, and reliability and validity of this measure as a diagnostic tool. It is stressed again that our purpose is to focus on documenting results within a report and not the "how" to administer many of these various techniques and their interpretations. If an evaluator is going to report these data, it is important that there be a full understanding of the measurement and the most reliable way to collect the data.

Basically described, a diadochokinetic rate is determined by asking the client or patient to rapidly produce a series of consonant-vowel syllables such as "papapapa" or "tatatata" or in a combination such as "pataka." The sounds are timed and the number of repetitions is counted to establish a number of syllables per second rate. There are different methods of assessment contributing to confusion in this area. Fletcher (1972) described a "typical" approach where the number of syllables produced in a given amount of time is counted. This is referred to as the count-by-time method. Fletcher further reports a time-by-count method where time needed to produce a determined number of syllables is measured. Hedge and Freed (2011) and Freed (2012) further clarify the idea in specifying the need to distinguish between the alternate motion rate, where alternating syllables are produced (pataka), and sequential motion rate, where single syllables are repeated (papapa). To aid in determining accurate data, it has been strongly suggested that this measure be recorded. Measurements determined are then compared to published diadochokinesis rates by age in published tables. These also vary. Given the limited research and controversy on the use of this measurement and varied methods in which data are collected and analyzed, it is cautioned that the evaluator be sure to review the available research to be able to report and document the use of diadochokinetic rates in the most reliable and evidence-based manner.

The manner in which the task was administered, how the rates were measured, the rates of production, stimuli used, and the comparison tables against which rates are assessed should be reported. If difficulties in task execution are noted, they should also be described, as they might be indicative of possible underlying oral motor deficits. These difficulties may include lack of breath support for the timed segment, variations in volume or pitch, difficulty in completing the task, or difficulty in actually sequencing varied monosyllable consonant-vowel productions. The limitations of the task as a standardized, objective measurement should be understood, and the evaluator should understand exactly what they are observing and what possible difficulties with this task mean. Again, as long as information is clearly documented and explained, it becomes useful to the reader and those using the final diagnostic report for a variety of reasons, including planning interventions, determining frequency and duration of therapy, and supporting funding of services.

REFERENCES

American Speech-Language-Hearing Association. (2016). *Scope of practice in speech language pathology.* https://www.asha.org/Policy/SP2016-00343/

Fletcher, S. G. (1972). Time-by-count measurement of diadochokinetic syllable rate. *Journal of Speech and Hearing Research, 15,* 763–770.

Freed, D. B. (2012). *Motor speech disorders: Diagnosis and treatment.* Delmar.

Hegde, M. N., & Freed, D. (2011). *Assessment of communication disorders in adults* (2nd ed.). Plural.

Chapter

8

Choosing the Language for Documenting Language

For the speech-language pathologist who is a "general practitioner" and evaluates clients or patients with a variety of disorders across a range of ages, most final written evaluations will have a significant section of the evaluation report devoted to the results of the language assessment. Evaluations of clients, usually children, referred for possible language delays, language disorders, specific language impairment, social pragmatic language disorders, and language-based learning disabilities, are not uncommon referrals for the majority of speech-language pathologists in school settings, agencies, and private practices. Diagnoses such as autism spectrum disorder and intellectual disability will also require thorough assessments of language functioning. Disorders and conditions requiring evaluation of language function will continue well through adolescence as academic or social challenges that were not necessarily evident at earlier ages and stages emerge. Evaluations are then recommended to rule out receptive, expressive, or pragmatic language issues as contributing factors. Trauma and acquired medical conditions that affect language function can occur at any age, and a speech and language evaluation will be necessary to assess the nature and severity of such disorders and provide recommendations for interventions. For children through adults, unless one specializes solely in a specific disorder such as voice, stuttering, or dysphagia, an analysis and description of some element of language function is associated with numerous underlying etiologies, conditions, and symptoms that will prompt a referral for assessing language as part of the evaluation.

Blaustein, S. H. *Diagnostic Report Writing in Speech-Language Pathology: A Guide to Effective Communication* (pp. 61-77).
© 2023 Taylor & Francis Group.

A Good Place to Start

In assessing the varied and complex aspects of language and then writing evaluation reports describing language function, clinicians typically rely heavily on norm-referenced standardized tests. These types of tests provide straightforward, relatively easy, and generally accepted ways to gather comparative data based on psychometric principles. These can be incorporated directly into a speech and language evaluation report and provide many advantages in evaluating language that clinicians should be well aware of. Evaluators should understand the difference between the term "standardized tests" and "standardized norm-referenced tests" as they do not mean the same thing. A standardized test will provide a "standard" procedure for test administration. The method of test administration is provided to ensure, as much as possible, that the test is administered in the same manner to all test takers. This is to ensure that the same materials and other stimuli, verbal and nonverbal, are presented to examinees to reduce variability in administration and differences in evaluators, as well as improve aspects of reliability. The goal is uniform test administration and scoring. A standardized norm-referenced test allows an individual's performance to be compared to an established group of peers. Through psychometric analysis of the test developer's results, scores are provided that allow for comparisons and variations in performance on a test to the average or mean performance of the group. Evaluators should be thoroughly familiar with these aspects and use of tests.

Standardized and/or standardized norm-referenced tests have specific age ranges associated with them. The number of tests, aspects of language assessed, and methods of scoring and interpretation are significant. This is especially true for individuals generally under 21 years of age. Numerous standardized assessments are available for older individuals with disorders such as aphasia, traumatic brain injury, or dementia, but for reasons not to be explained here, results are more task, function, criterion, or classification based. Standardized norm-referenced tests are available for adults, but numbers and variety are more limited. Each type of standardized assessment used by an evaluator will not only require an understanding of its specific manner of administration but will also require its own specific manner of reporting, analysis, interpretation, and documentation. This will be specified in each examiner's manual that accompanies each test published and purchased.

It is in the "Language" section of the diagnostic report that the examiner's results of norm-referenced standardized assessments, standardized assessments, criterion-referenced assessments, authentic assessments, and dynamic assessments must be clearly presented, described, and explained. The results will be analyzed and used to determine whether or not a delay, disorder, or deficit in language is a contributing component to the individual's presenting problem. Results may also determine if a language problem is related to a specific diagnosis and what recommendations and referrals are needed.

Dealing With the Complexities of Reporting Language Assessment

If one were to visit the exhibit hall at an annual national convention of the American Speech-Language-Hearing Association, it would be hard not to be overwhelmed by the number of publishers in attendance exhibiting literally hundreds of standardized tests and materials that are marketed toward speech-language pathologists for use in assessments and evaluations. This presentation is in addition to the multiple regular mailings of catalogues and frequent emails from publishers further promoting available tests by category. The vast number and variety of language tests available, specific purposes and objectives of each test, types of information elicited, differences in scoring methodology from test to test, the specific vocabulary that each test developer uses to designate the subtests and indices, and the test developer's description of interpretation and analysis of results are all multiplied by the numbers of available tests. The competent evaluator must thoroughly be aware of test purposes, content, and availability in the areas they assess and be able to select each of the appropriate tests that will provide needed information to best determine a patient's or client's level of functioning in the areas called for based on the presenting problem or problems. That is only half of the ultimate challenge to the evaluator. Once the evaluation is complete, the speech-language pathologist must then be able to organize and clearly present the findings, analysis, and interpretation of the language assessment in a written diagnostic report so that others may benefit from their results. The examiner must be able to explain to the reader what language assessment measures were used, why they were selected, and the information learned from their administration. The various scoring categories, comparison of categories, and information obtained within individual tests and between tests must be discussed. Results of standard tests must be viewed along with results of authentic assessments and other measures to determine congruence or disparity in performance in areas assessed, and if so, why? All of this must be included in written form in the diagnostic report. There is little available standardized or evidence-based information on the optimal and most efficient manner in which this should be accomplished.

As difficult and complex as this may appear, there is a logical approach to documenting the language section within the evaluation. As is seen throughout this book, there is a basic format to the way assessments are planned. This is largely determined by the reason for referral, age of the individual to be assessed, and case history. That information will then provide the blueprint for the specific tests selected and other assessments that will initially be administered. Writing the report is analogous to following the blueprint and describing the end result.

Knowing just the age of the individual to be assessed immediately excludes, and allows, any number of tests to be selected that are generally standardized and limited by age range. Knowing additional information about client backgrounds, additional languages spoken or exposed to, and limitations in attention, vision, writing, restricted manual dexterity, or hearing might also preclude or include tests based on specific requirements and standardization criteria specified within each test. The evaluator then must carefully consider the nature of the language difficulties, problems or challenges to be assessed as they were presented in the referral, and case history. What possible problems in language areas are called into question? If it is understanding or comprehension, is it following directions, understanding stories, following discourse, or difficulty with vocabulary or memory? If it is expressive language, is it organization, word finding, morphology, or sequencing stories? Difficulties may be related to pragmatic language areas such as topic maintenance or recognizing listeners' needs. Whatever the reasons for referral and evaluation, the examiner, in order to properly assess any possible areas of difficulty, must plan an initial assessment test battery to begin to determine any underlying areas of weakness or deficit that would explain the questioned difficulty or rule out areas of language as contributing factors. Strengths must also be assessed. Eventually, this must be explained in the written evaluation.

What is clear from this discussion is that a broad knowledge of available tests and measurements, as well as their objectives, uses, and basic properties, is essential for the speech-language pathologist who chooses to serve as a diagnostician. One needs not only to have current knowledge of the vast variety of tests available but also to have access to current versions, associated test forms and materials, and the time and ability to administer enough of the assessments that would permit full analysis and interpretation for diagnosis and documentation. Unfortunately, there are many barriers to this occurring, and they may become evident in the final evaluation reports produced. Some of these barriers warrant a brief discussion as challenges to be taken into consideration before one chooses to conduct an evaluation of language function. Many of these same limitations will apply to other areas being assessed where tests are required. These areas include:

1. **Lack of knowledge or experience.** Many evaluators are limited to administering only the tests they learned in graduate training. There is a level of comfort and familiarity that one does not move beyond. One who chooses to evaluate must read the journals, take continuing education courses in assessment and diagnosis, and keep up with all of the publishers catalogues that are received that offer tests, updates, new tests, and tests continuing to be published. Be aware of tests that are no longer published or available and why.

2. **Lack of access.** Evaluators may be employed in settings that due to budgetary, space, or other concerns do not purchase or provide the wide array of tests that are necessary for thorough evaluation. Many times, the latest versions of tests may not be available. This also applies to evaluators in private practice who limit necessary test purchases.

3. **Time constraints.** It takes varying amounts of time to complete an assessment based on the complexity of the case or response rate of the patient or client. For certain conditions, hours of testing may be called for. Evaluators may have self- or externally imposed time restrictions allowed for evaluations.

4. **Limited commitment to assessments.** Evaluating speech and language disorders requires a commitment that involves time, resources, and knowledge and experience. For clinicians who primarily provide therapy and do the occasional assessment, realize that the assessment is as important as, if not more important than, the therapy and requires a high level of expertise, experience, time, and resources. Do not accept referrals for evaluations where there is not experience, appropriate testing materials, and a full understanding of all elements required for the evaluation of a specific disorder.

Any one or combination of these limitations may hamper a thorough assessment of language function. In fact, any aspect of speech, language, or communication functioning assessment will be limited if the evaluator is not fully committed to the assessment process with time, materials, and knowledge. The documented results of any evaluation can only be as complete as the results generated by the process itself. This is particularly true for the complexities of describing a patient's or client's use of language.

How to Document Test Results: Just Describe What You Did

There is a way to plan, proceed with, and complete a language evaluation. Documenting results should logically follow the assessment process. Necessary information should be presented in a clear and logical format that will facilitate the writing process. Mastering this process can then generalize from report to report. Experience will facilitate writing. Each report produced will be easier to complete than the previous one as a result of what was previously learned about the process itself.

A clinician usually begins a general language assessment with an omnibus language test that contains selected targeted subtests that will initially evaluate and provide data concerning the problems in question relative to the reason for the referral. An omnibus test refers to a specific type of test or assessment that will evaluate a variety of abilities, in this case related to language, during the same administration as part of the same test. One single omnibus test, for example, can be administered to test numerous aspects of receptive language, expressive language, and even pragmatics. There are many such tests to choose from, and this is where the evaluator's knowledge and experience will come into play. Each omnibus assessment has its own specific subtests, areas assessed, and ways to score, interpret, and use test results. The evaluator, based on the referral and case history, will select a certain test to begin with as a result of having specific knowledge and experience with an omnibus assessment previously used, read about, or learned about in a presentation or workshop. With experience, just the nature of the referral will automatically trigger the name of a specific test to start with. In many omnibus language tests, there are individual test scores from subtests that measure discrete areas of language that can stand alone and be reported without the need to administer the complete omnibus test. How subtests from an omnibus test are used and whether or not they can be used and reported individually is information that will be included in the examiner's manual. An entire omnibus test therefore need not be administered. If the evaluator would like one specific area of language to be assessed, there are omnibus tests that allow for administration of multiple identified discrete subtests that yield an index score or core score. The individual subtest scores are combined and analysis of a few tests in certain areas yields information about wider areas of function. These "index" scores can then be used to assess broader areas within language such as memory, phonological awareness, receptive language, expressive language, or pragmatics. These subarea scores can be further used to determine greater insight into the patient's overall functioning. Results can be compared between index scores to determine relative areas of specific weakness or strength, which will lead to planning for additional assessments. This is often referred to as a discrepancy analysis. This all serves as part of what is termed a differential diagnosis, that is, helping determine what something is by establishing what it is not. Evaluators should be familiar with all of these areas of assessing language briefly summarized here.

The examiner, based on the initial results of an omnibus test, may then select to administer additional specific targeted tests. Similarly, the results may indicate that there are areas that are stronger and need no or limited further testing. This is also part of using a differential diagnosis. Further language areas are then explored, assessed, and eventually understood. Additional tests administered may also include other omnibus-type tests, but of a more narrow range. Omnibus tests are available that assess a specific narrower aspect of language but that can still be viewed considering a number of different skills related to that area that should be assessed. These may simultaneously assess skills of auditory processing, vocabulary, narrative production, or pragmatics to gain further insight into an individual's areas of strength and weakness. These additional assessments will have a rationale for administration and continue to provide additional information that will hopefully enable the evaluator to address the questions raised in the original reason for the referral.

The evaluator should also be knowledgeable about the numerous assessment instruments available that, unlike the omnibus assessments, test a very limited range or one specific skill. As the evaluator continues with the assessment, analyzes the results, and gets more of an understanding through a client's or patient's performance in the various areas, the scope of testing gets more and more specific to allow the evaluator to narrow down possible areas of difficulty and have information to document these results. There are numerous tests targeted to single areas available that include receptive vocabulary, expressive vocabulary, auditory discrimination, understanding and use of paragraphs, word finding, and problem solving, just to name a few. With respect to standardized testing, this is generally how the language evaluation occurs, develops, and grows from the consolidated information learned from the selected tests administered as the evaluation proceeds. This must all eventually be competently and clearly documented.

The procedure for conducting an evaluation results in a series of steps through testing that result in gathering data that will eventually be used to analyze, synthesize, and document the final results and determinations. Understanding the reason for the referral, important information gleaned from the case history, and then using an omnibus testing and getting more and more specific as discrete skills are evaluated will enable the evaluator to begin to understand a client's overall functioning and answer the question regarding the reason for the referral and the difficulties with functional skills that usually prompted the referral. Realizing the approach that is suggested for the standardized part of the language assessment can enable one to appreciate the skill, experience, and access to the resources necessary to complete an evaluation. Unfortunately, there are times when an individual evaluator may stop short of the depth and breadth needed for complete assessment, and decisions may therefore be based on limited underlying diagnostic support. Unless sufficient results are thorough, complete, carefully interpreted, filtered, and properly applied, confusion can arise in the final evaluation report. Such confusion in a final written document may not stand up to review or scrutiny of sophisticated questioning or analysis. This may result in incorrect diagnosis or the loss of services, placement, or necessary referrals a client or patient may be seeking.

CHARTS HELP

In dealing with the wide range and types of scores an individual test can yield, it must be understood that the data from each test must be organized, presented, and discussed. Since the vast majority of reports will include language assessment results from multiple tests as the results of all standardized assessments, scores derived must be included in the report. They should be presented as a group somewhere in the report in chart form. This may be included as an appendix following the report or presented as its own section, preferably at the beginning of the report. A complete list of tests and scores in one place allows the reader to get an initial idea of the tests used, ranges of scores, comparisons of scores, and extent of testing. Organizing a complete list of tests and scores will also assist the evaluator in organizing their thoughts, determining order of presentation within the report, and aiding in the eventual narrative presentation. Viewing a complete list and summary of all test scores allows for a concise and uncluttered view of relative areas of strength and weakness and ensures that all tests administered are included. The hypothetical results of a popular omnibus test, the Clinical Evaluation of Language Fundamentals-5 (Wiig et al., 2013), from one administration for one individual are presented in chart form as an example. Table 8-1 presents an example of how test results might be presented in simple chart form. Some of the varied types of useful standardized norm-referenced scores obtainable are included in the chart for illustrative purposes. The name of the test and each of the individual subtests is evident. It is noted that the subtest scores are scaled scores. Equivalent percentile scores from the conversion table in the examiner's manual are also present. Confidence intervals and raw scores for each subtest are available but have not been included to simplify the chart. The experienced examiner will be aware that age scores, grade scores, and growth scores are also available but have not been included. Each has their own limitation and purpose and can be included at the examiner's discretion. Charts can be developed based on each test and the evaluator's preferences and specific reporting needs.

The table presented lists the index scores that can be generated. They allow comparison of wider areas of language ability conceptualized by the test authors that have been psychometrically compiled by combining selected, relevant, theoretically related subtests. Note that these are presented as standard scores unlike the previous scaled scores for the subtests. The standard scores are labeled accordingly and are indicated in the table with the heading to indicate these are standard scores. The mean of 100 with a standard deviation of ±15 is also present. The test also allows for comparison of index scores (indices) to determine if there is a statistically significant difference between language areas assessed. The chart presented shows significant differences. In this case, it also states that one comparison is significant at the .05 level. Similar test results for each additional test administered would then continue to be provided in one summary table, and the test results can functionally be seen as an entire data set.

The evaluator must be aware of the types of scores available, which will vary from test to test. Understanding these scores, which ones to select, how they are interpreted and used, and, eventually, how to write about them in the final diagnostic report requires a skill set that a competent evaluator must possess. Once acquired, it is a basic theoretical tool box that will serve the clinician well and will only improve with experience. Knowing how to present and use the data to understand a patient or client, support a diagnosis, defend a report, and advocate to qualify for programs, services, or reimbursement makes for a successful and sought-after language evaluator.

TABLE 8-1		
Example of Chart to Report Norm-Referenced Scoring		
CLINICAL EVALUATION OF LANGUAGE FUNDAMENTALS-5		
Subtest	*Scaled Score*	*Percentile*
Word Classes	6	9
Following Directions	4	2
Formulated Sentences	11	63
Recalling Sentences	10	50
Understanding Spoken Paragraphs	6	9
Word Definitions	7	16
Sentence Assembly	9	37
Semantic Relationships	9	37
(mean = 10; SD = ±3)		
CORE LANGUAGE AND INDEX SCORES		
	Standard Score	*Percentile*
Core Language Score	93	32
Receptive Language Index	82	12
Expressive Language Index	100	50
Language Content Index	82	12
Language Memory Index	90	25
(mean = 100; SD = ±15)		
Index Discrepancy Comparisons		
Receptive-Expressive Language Index: Significant difference at .05 level		
Language Content-Memory Index: No significant difference		

A Chart Is Not Enough

A chart provided within an evaluation, however helpful and complete, cannot remain in isolation. As meaningful as they might be, they are just scores. The content of the tests and additional information concerning the tests administered must be described and discussed in the body of the report. This will allow for a fuller understanding of what the patient or client was asked to do, how they performed, and what the results were in context. This information will be later used as part of the final analysis of the individual's functioning to provide the summary and impressions, as well as support a diagnosis.

When writing evaluation reports, clinicians often rely heavily, when age appropriate, on norm-referenced standardized assessments. They provide a straightforward, relatively easy, and accepted way to access comparative data that can be incorporated directly into a speech and language evaluation report and provide the many advantages that evaluators are generally aware of. Given the complexities and variations in norm-referenced standardized assessments and criterion-based assessments, it is incumbent on the test administrator and diagnostic report writer to fully understand every element of the test they are using and the information provided, including the administration, scoring, interpretations, and strengths and weaknesses of each test selected. Much of this information, if relevant, is referenced in the eventual written language assessment. It stands to reason that the test administrator should be aware of this information to be an accountable and skilled tester; a clear understanding of the test instruments administered will make description of the test in the final written evaluations more meaningful to the users. All of the basic and advanced information regarding specific tests and their administration can be obtained in the examiner's manual. The evaluator should be familiar with the information as much of it can be incorporated into the final report to aid in documentation, explanation, and accountability. Careful and skilled use of psychometric principles, test purposes, scoring, and interpretation as specified in examiner's manuals will add increased credibility to an evaluator's written presentation. All published, recognized standardized tests purchased contain an examiner's manual, as well as may contain a technical manual, instructions to administer the test, scoring tables, stimuli, and test protocols. Tests also provide test stimuli in the form of pictures or actual objects, toys, or manipulatives that are necessary to administer the test. Understanding all of these elements is critical. It must be noted that an increasing number of speech and language tests are now available in digital platforms for computer, remote, and telepractice administration. The evaluator is cautioned to carefully read the examiners manual to determine standardization characteristics and appropriateness of reporting norm-referenced results.

What Else to Write

The previous discussion described omnibus tests, using test performance to guide additional test selection, types of scores derived, and how a clinician might simply present them in a chart format. It is necessary to also include a narrative section where more detailed information will be presented about the test results and further information will be provided to clarify for the reader what the test scores reported actually represent. In the narrative language section, the goal is to succinctly discuss the tests administered, the scores, and what the scores reported represent. Examples of incorrect responses may be included to allow the reader to understand the nature of the difficulty the individual may be experiencing with various language tasks. It must be remembered that as part of the final analysis, using the language scores reported in addition to all of the other relevant information gathered from the assessment process will be synthesized and discussed in the summary and impression sections of the report. The language assessment results will be used in determining the critical decisions of diagnosis, severity, and whatever recommendations and referrals must be made.

An important question that an evaluator should continue to ask is who will ultimately be reading and using the report being generated. Speech-language pathologists will likely only be a small percentage of the readers. Pediatricians, neurologists, psychologists, teachers, administrators, reviewers for insurance companies, participants in Early Intervention, Committee on Preschool Special Education members, Committee on Special Education members, and parents are examples of the ultimate readers and users of the reports speech-language pathologists write. In the era of Interprofessional Practice, an ever widening and varied group of professionals will be asked to consider, use, and discuss the information provided in our reports. Results of standardized language assessments and evaluating a variety of specific linguistic functions can be difficult for a reader unfamiliar with the language concepts and terms described to fully grasp. While we must continue to write professionally, in the manner we were trained, we must also consider that the information must be functional and understandable to outside readers. The technical jargon we use, familiarity with common tests that are published and administered, abbreviations, interpretations of the results, and even diagnostic impressions may be unfamiliar to most readers of our reports. A report should therefore be user-friendly, remembering that if the report is not functional to the reader, its utility is greatly diminished. An evaluator, in the written language assessment narrative, can use a professional lexicon but should also strive to present results through careful clinical presentation discussed in a user-friendly way. There have been numerous times when this author has been asked to arrange for a consultation to review and explain the results of a speech and language evaluation to a parent or family. Even after a review by the original evaluator, parents, family, clients, or patients still have questions, misunderstanding, or confusion about what was done and the results. This should not have to occur with a well-written report and appropriate follow-up meeting to discuss results.

What elements should then be considered in presenting standardized norm-referenced language test results? To begin with, the name of the test should be clearly and completely stated. Too often, diagnostic reports are written where only abbreviations are used. These abbreviations, although common to speech-language pathologists, are unfamiliar to most readers and, in fact, may be unfamiliar to many speech-language pathologists. Begin by stating the complete name of the test. If an abbreviation is to be used, include it in parentheses immediately following the initial naming of the test, for example, Clinical Evaluation of Language Fundamentals-5 (CELF-5). Note the "5" in the previous example. This indicates that the fifth revision of the test was utilized. It is extremely important to indicate which version of a test is being used. A second publication of a test may be indicated with "-R." This is indicative of a revision. Tests may then continue to be revised and updated, and subsequent revisions are then usually numbered as 3, 4, and so on. Each of these tests is different. They are updated and contain changes, response to criticisms from test users, new statistical data that improve scoring, and other critical changes that are specific to the test as identified by the specific name. It should also be remembered that the latest and most recent available published edition of a test should be used. Using an older version of a test when a newer one is available raises questions about the data and the expertise of the evaluator.

Following providing the exact name of the test administered, a short statement describing the purpose of the test is helpful. This brief explanation of the purpose of a test can be useful for any reader. For example, if a test is designed to evaluate an individual's understanding of single-item vocabulary, then state that "the ABC Test was administered to assess the ability to identify single-item receptive vocabulary from an auditory prompt." The score then provided will be all the more meaningful as the reader understands what ability the score represents. Many other tests that will be administered may also assess just one specific aspect of language production. It is not difficult to learn to state the functions of these specifically targeted tests administered as evaluating expressive vocabulary, word retrieval, or ability to follow directions or label pictures presented. The purpose, objectives, or goals of a test are always specified in the examiner's manual and may be quoted directly if properly referenced. Test users should be thoroughly familiar with all of the components contained in a standardized test and be certain to read all manuals, review all stimulus material, and understand scoring protocols. It is critical that if an examiner chooses a specific test to administer in their evaluation, they should be fully aware of all aspects of the selected assessment instrument. This will not only be helpful in fully appreciating and understanding the test used but assist the clinician in determining which relevant information to include in the narrative and summary sections. Inclusion of various scores, their derivation, and interpretation related to language function can prove effective in completing more properly supported and documented evaluations. Much of the information made available by publishers to test users will also serve to provide accountability and rationale for test selection if the choice is ever questioned. Information on scoring, interpretation, standardization samples, specificity, and sensitivity, among other factors, may often be included in evaluation reports obtained in the examiner's manual. Table 8-2 provides a list of information frequently available in an examiner's manual. Many evaluators, perhaps to save time, will become familiar with how a test is administered and scored and avoid a full review of the examiner's manual. Much information is lost, and this loss can easily be reflected in how test results are used and documented in the final report. Evaluators should also be aware of Burrows Mental Measurement Yearbook, which is a nationally recognized publication of available tests in numerous disciplines, including speech-language pathology. Basic information regarding each test is provided along with critiques of each test. This can be helpful in test selection and in purchasing and evaluating tests.

In continuing to document test results and to provide a greater understanding of the results of the test, it is helpful to specify what the client or patient is asked to do. For example, it may be stated that the client was asked to point to one picture, from an array of four, that matches (or best describes) the word stated by the examiner. In more straightforward assessments that largely assess one general area of language function, the reader will then understand prior to presenting a result the name of the test, the purpose of the test, and what the client or patient was asked to do. This provides a greater understanding to the reader of what the score provided represents.

TABLE 8-2
Useful Information Contained in Examiner's Manual for Documentation

• Description of test	• Test standardization
• Purpose of test	• Test development
• Administration guidelines	• Test components
• Scoring instructions	• Administration time
• Test reliability and validity	• Examiner qualifications
• Theoretical basis of test	• Cultural/dialectal variables
• Interpreting test scores	• Curriculum-related details
• Types of scores	• Relevant research
• Score conversion tables	• Accommodations and modifications

Many tests are much more complicated than simply having one or even two straightforward aspects of language to assess. Tests are developed by researchers, clinicians, faculty, and others who work from a conceptual understanding of aspects of language and seek to develop assessment instruments that assess these aspects as important underlying skills that can be measured. Results lead to understanding language performance within a test author's theoretical framework. Within a specified framework, results allow the evaluator to identify areas of possible language weaknesses or strength. All of this information is helpful in diagnosing or recognizing an underlying disorder, and these are essential components in determining recommendations.

Let's suppose, then, that a test developer determines that assessing single-item receptive vocabulary is not sufficient in understanding an individual's vocabulary comprehension. A test developer might decide there is more utility and validity in assessing vocabulary if many aspects of vocabulary can be differentiated. Thus, a vocabulary test may assess the comprehension of nouns, verbs, categorical items, and descriptors. They may further be able to specify and delineate certain words that describe temporal or quantitative concepts. The scoring of the test may then be developed to provide subtest scores that allow an understanding of an individual's performance in each of these subareas and also can provide an overall total vocabulary score. These subtleties and complexities in test design must be explained to the reader for clarification. It will allow the reader to have a greater understanding of language function in the individual being assessed. Thus, to describe the purpose of a more detailed test, more of a description is needed, a statement such as "The ABC Total Vocabulary Test assesses the comprehension of single-item vocabulary and further allows for the ability to differentiate and assess receptive vocabulary comprehension into discrete areas such as nouns, verbs, and descriptors." While a description of how the test is administered may remain the same, the information yielded differs with relevant subtest and total scores available. These scores will eventually be provided in the report, and the reader will have a greater understanding of how they were elicited and what they mean. The previous example describes how receptive vocabulary may be divided into delineated areas, but there are larger, more comprehensive tests that can separate broader areas such as receptive language, expressive language, memory, pragmatics, and so on. This must also be described and scores attained must be provided.

Describing Even More Specific Types of Scores

Many test developers seeking to maximize their assessment instrument, philosophy, or conceptual understanding of components of language and ability to analyze an individual's language performance may develop a more varied and comprehensive assessment instrument. This is usually in the form of the omnibus test previously described. They provide a number of varied and useful scores that have been determined based on psychometric principles that allow greater understanding of an individual's test performance. If these scores are available, they must be provided to the reader and described briefly. They will also be used by the evaluator in a final analysis and used in the summary and impression, to support a greater understanding of an individual's language function. Referencing these scores and describing them earlier in the report will set the stage for their inclusion in a final analytic discussion.

The scope of this text is not to provide an in-depth understanding of test scoring, psychometric principles, or test selection. For the purposes of diagnostic report writing, it is important to understand the breadth and depth of scores that are available and must be understood and documented. Readers unfamiliar with these scores should seek further study as they are common in many tests currently utilized by speech-language pathologists. Understanding these scores will not only ultimately assist in writing a final diagnostic report but are also critical in test selection, administration, scoring, analysis, interpretation, and final recommendations. Without a full understanding of the objectives of a test, scoring, and what the scores derived represent, the client or patient is not best served and the best evidence-based practice remains at risk. Furthermore, unless the clinician understands the principles discussed, there is no way a truly valid report will be produced. Scores reported should be described. A few of these common scores will be discussed as they might be described in a report.

Index scores or indices represent a number or score that, based on psychometric principles, represent the composite results of a number of selected subtests within a test. Subtests are grouped to provide scores to assess performance in broader areas of function. Subtest scores can be combined in a manner that enables assessment of areas such as memory, receptive language, or expressive language. This concept was previously discussed. When reporting an index score, the clinician should briefly state what an index score represents, the broader area being assessed, the subtests involved, and what the results were. Some tests also enable the clinician using index scores to compare scores statistically to determine how great the degree of differences between skill areas measured within a test actually are. The difference between two index scores can be compared using Discrepancy Scoring Tables provided by test developers to determine not only if the difference in scores is significant but also at what level of significance this occurs. The clinician can also choose to provide what percentage of the standardization sample scored the discrepancy level. These scores can be helpful in analyzing performance, describing strengths and weaknesses, determining goals, and making recommendations to individuals we assess who are experiencing communication disorders. Thus, an individual attaining a scaled score of 7 on receptive language and a scaled score of 6 or 8 on expressive language might not indicate a statistically significant discrepancy. Yet a scaled score of 10 in receptive language and a scaled score of 4 in expressive language may be indicative of a significant relative weakness in one area. These data must be understood, described, explained, and provided. The following statement is an example of how discussion of an index score may be included in a report. The basic interpretation of the index score results will then be incorporated within the summary and impressions section to provide an understanding of overall language function and assist in determining a diagnosis. The results of the index scores presented in Table 8-1 are used in this example.

The Clinical Evaluation of Language Fundamentals-5 combines selected subtest scores to provide index scores to determine test performance in selected, broader areas of language function. William attained a Receptive Language Index at the 12th percentile (SS = 82) and an Expressive Language Index at the 50th percentile (SS = 100). While both index scores fall at or below the 50th percentile, the 18-point standard score difference is significant at the .05 level. This degree of difference occurred in only 4.6% of the normative sample.

Receptive language is shown to be a relatively weaker area of language function for William according to test interpretation. No statistically significant difference was found between the Language Content Index (SS = 82) and Language Memory Index (SS = 90).

One other example of a score that is frequently reported in results of standardized language sections is a confidence interval. Within each test that we administer and score, there is allowance for a standard error of measurement. Individuals may vary in their test-taking abilities, and there may be some variance in the way tests are administered. This occurs even though tests are standardized in an effort to reduce variability. The confidence interval measurement allows a statistical prediction of how an individual will score on repeated administrations of the same test, allowing for variations in performance or administration. The ability to determine this confidence interval is often specified at the 90th or 95th percent level of confidence. The level can be determined by the test administrator by selecting the desired level in the test's conversion chart. A test evaluator who determines that an individual has a standard score of 100 at the 50th percentile can then find confidence interval numbers specified in the test manual. This may be stated as ±8, ±15 and so on. Thus, although an individual attained a standard score of 100 on a particular test administration, it could be stated in the report that the confidence interval at the 95th percentile would be ±8 and vary from a standard score of 92 to a standard score of 108. The corresponding percentiles would vary from the 30th percentile to the 70th percentile. Specifying the confidence intervals provides greater use of each individual test's psychometric and statistical properties and also provides additional understanding to an informed reader. One must be diligent in reporting results in that a variety of test scores are frequently provided by the test developers for different uses within the same test. The scores must be utilized, reported, and discussed correctly. It is critical to recognize the types of scores used and not make errors on reporting these numbers. It is up to the examiner to decide which scores to include in the final document, realizing which are required and essential and additional scores that may be supplementary.

Standardized language assessment is an important factor in evaluating language. Clinicians should be aware of the benefits and disadvantages of using such assessments. Whenever they are used, it is important that the clinician is aware of the nature of the assessment, scores derived, and, as importantly, how to interpret and document the results of their use. While tests vary in many ways, there is also a great deal of uniformity in the types of scores produced, terminology for these scores, and even their interpretation. Knowing this will allow the clinician to become more comfortable, efficient, flexible, and confident in writing the language section of the evaluation report.

DOCUMENTING AUTHENTIC LANGUAGE ASSESSMENTS

Disruptions in both receptive and expressive language and pragmatics occur in numerous congenital, developmental, and acquired disorders and conditions. They may vary in their severity and impact on functional, academic, and social manifestations. A key responsibility within the scope of practice of speech-language pathologists is to assess language ability across the life span for clients and patients. Thorough assessment and reporting of language function is accomplished in numerous ways and requires the skill set of knowing the areas of language to assess and the specific standardized and authentic measures to use based on the nature of the referral. Once again, the task becomes not only to complete the appropriate evaluation and possible diagnosis but to then report and document the results in a clear and efficient manner. This must be done for both the standardized and authentic measures. Authentic assessments are becoming increasingly more critical in evaluating individuals from culturally and linguistically diverse backgrounds who are often not represented in the standardization samples of many norm-referenced tests available.

It has been discussed that standardized assessments by their nature, design, and function lend themselves to a more straightforward and therefore easier reporting of results. The process of norm-referenced standardization provides psychometric data that can include raw scores, percentiles, standard or scaled scores (or both), confidence intervals, index scores, and, in some cases, discrepancy comparisons that are determined by an individual's performance.

Authentic testing, often referred to as informal or spontaneous assessment, is considerably more difficult to document. Unlike standardized norm-referenced assessments that are clear, data driven, and specific in their results, the informal assessment is overtly more subjective. In this type of assessment, the evaluator seeks to gain additional information about the client or patient through eliciting a more "natural" communication that more mirrors the everyday demands and challenges of language use. Authentic testing has many advantages, must be used in our assessments, and provides a great deal of diagnostic information. Unlike standardized testing, however, authentic testing varies from evaluator to evaluator, client to client, and patient to patient and is solely dependent upon the skill, expertise, and decisions made by the clinician conducting the assessment. Following formal standardized assessments, areas of weakness and strength are determined and decisions are made as to how to further probe specific language areas. These decisions will also be based on the reason for referral and case history information. A variety of planned tasks, questions, discourse, play, observations, and language challenges are used in informal assessments. These will vary greatly based on the information desired. The ability to plan these tasks around the client or patient with knowledge of the specific information about language function needed is just one of the advantages of an informal assessment. The evaluator may also seek to probe language use beyond the traditional and somewhat limited therapy office setting. An evaluator can decide that a language sample is needed from a classroom, playground, lunchroom, home, office space, or telephone conversation. The setting for collecting a language sample becomes an additional factor in the assessment. Less available are specific guidelines on how these findings should be documented in our reports. Most standardized assessments will include a section in the examiner's test manual describing the ideal "environment" to conduct the assessment, yet an explanation of the authentic environment is left up to the individual evaluator. Authentic assessment is accomplished in a variety of settings, which are required by the nature of this type of measurement. The setting of the assessment must be clearly specified.

As one continues to understand the nature of the authentic assessment, a series of considerations or processes appears. Like other aspects of the evaluation, these processes follow a logical order and are based on a knowledge and understanding of the components of an evaluation, and although disorders and symptoms will vary, the basic conceptual framework for what the evaluator needs to accomplish is quite similar from etiology to etiology and individual to individual. This holds true for the diagnostic evaluation report that follows each assessment. The elements, general areas of content, what and how to document, and even order of presentation of results remain very similar. Appreciating these facts leads to the understanding that report writing is a systems-based process that follows an ordered and logical progression that has a strong degree of similarity in the nature of the task. Yes, there will be a different report for every client and patient, but the processes, steps, and even final look and order of the document will be very similar.

As we continue to discuss authentic assessment, another variable that must be considered is the goal of this part of the evaluation. This becomes another important factor to document and include in any language narrative report. Authentic assessment can be used to provide additional insights into overall intelligibility of speech, comprehension, expressive language, word retrieval, attention, pragmatics, or working memory, just to name a few possible targets. These will be the areas that have been determined by the results of the standardized testing or reported areas of concern indicated in the reason for referral. All of this must also be well specified and documented in the final clinical report. In determining the goal of the authentic assessment(s), the description of the setting and context must be provided. This includes reporting the individuals involved in the communication interactions. This frequently involves others beyond solely the clinician. It is critical to interpret and understand language use "in the moment," how the language "use" targeted for assessment was used by the individual in that particular setting in that moment, who the participants were, and the nature of the language demands. Without this background, even if briefly stated, the reader will have little idea of the levels and appropriateness of the language being understood and produced. A transcription of a dialogue or narrative without context will be much less meaningful.

TABLE 8-3
Authentic Language Assessment Elements and Examples

CONSIDERATION	EXAMPLE
Goal of assessment	To assess following directions, word retrieval, language initiation, topic maintenance
Approach	Classroom observation, simulation, language sample, video review
Specific measures	Mean length of utterance, type-token ratio, Systematic Analysis of Language Transcripts
Task	Block building, play game, phone call, take a message, reading lesson
Setting	Home, school, office, playground, park, restaurant
Participants	Teacher, peer(s), therapist, family members
Specific examples	Provide details of receptive/expressive language, social pragmatic, sound production areas that illustrate strength and weakness

Specifying the goal of the authentic assessment(s), specific environment, and activity taking place and participants sets the stage for understanding the ever-changing communication demands and how our client or patient responds to those demands. Specific examples must be provided, and how the information is interpreted must also be explained.

Specific examples, both strengths and weaknesses, that clearly illustrate the language performance of the individual being evaluated should be documented. They must be described within the context of the ever-varying demands of language. Often a transcript, or segment of a transcript, will be included in the actual document. If a longer utterance is elicited, such as in assessing narrative or expository speech, the examples may include the entire transcript or a number of paragraphs that clearly indicate the responses and enable the reader to understand the elements of the analysis that are selected for review. They should always be provided within a context and setting that allows for a greater understanding of the individual's use of language.

Once the sample has been described within the specific context, the evaluator must then analyze and interpret the specifically targeted language samples using sufficient information to support a final diagnostic impression. It is important to remember here that any authentic language tasks selected for this section of the evaluation are entirely up to the individual evaluator's discretion. The techniques, measures, tasks and rubrics, or means for assessing these tasks are entirely up to the skill, knowledge, and experience of the evaluator, reason for referral, and specific questions to be answered. Those questions will not be answered here. The determination and use of many of the subjective techniques used are both the strengths and weaknesses of this type of assessment. The common consideration, however, across all authentic assessments utilized is to be sure that the procedures and results are well documented. Table 8-3 summarizes elements of an authentic assessment that must be documented and provides examples for each element.

Many authentic measurement techniques are available, and graduate students and clinicians should be well aware of language sample analysis techniques. Some of these include type-token ratio, which provides a ratio of the variety of words in a sample to the total number of words in a collected sample. Mean length of utterance is a measure that determines the average number of morphemes per utterance in a series of utterances will generally correspond to a child's chronological age in typically developing children. Investigators continue to describe methods to facilitate language sample analysis, and the Narrative Assessment Protocol-2 (Bowles et al., 2020) is an example of a recently described assessment tool for evaluating language samples from video recordings of young children (ages 3 to 6 years), which is reported to be a psychometrically sound way to assess young children's narrative productions. While this technique is a standardized measure, it fills the gap to provide an additional measure of language sample analysis in an area where there are limited evidence-based techniques available. There are also computer-based language analysis programs such as Systematic Analysis of Language Transcripts (2022) and Sampling Utterances and Grammatical Analysis Revised (Owens & Pavelco, 2017). These computer-based language analysis programs are readily available and make the tedious job of analyzing language samples easier for the busy clinician. One can see from a brief description of some of the measures used to assess children's language that they are very specific, require knowledge and training in their use, and will involve a discipline-specific lexical base to understand exactly what aspects of language are measured and how they are interpreted. Less available are specific guidelines on how these findings should be documented in our reports to allow the lay individual to understand our findings.

Authentic assessments are also utilized in a variety of acquired language disorders such as aphasia, dementia, and traumatic brain injury. The assessment techniques are not as specific as those utilized in children, but nonetheless it is important to describe the functional impact of language loss across the life span. This should also be well documented in our language reports to allow for intervention planning, securing appropriate placements as needed, seeking reimbursement for services, and establishing very important baseline measures. The way these authentic measures are observed, collected, measured, and interpreted will vary with the disorder and clinician selection, which is why it is so important to accurately document them if used. The final authentic assessment must be written in consideration of the standardized assessment results, and the entire assessment, both standardized and informal, must be cohesive, make sense, be well analyzed, and eliminate or at least minimize any potential areas of dispute. In standardized assessment, one may question the use of a specific test. The results, however, stand by themselves. In authentic assessment, the tasks, environment, and results interpretation more readily lend themselves to criticism and dispute. One must therefore be exceedingly careful.

If an evaluator has a clear rationale for the authentic techniques used and can specify the specific parameters of the assessment along with the results and conclusions, it is a critical and important piece of the evaluation and subsequent final written diagnostic report. Due to the inherent subjective nature of authentic/informal evaluation, any authentic language tasks selected are entirely up to the individual evaluator's discretion. Missing elements or confusion in presentation can result in the reader, or ultimate user of the report, to raise questions, challenge assumptions made, lose confidence in the evaluator, find inconsistencies, or discount results. It is well accepted that an evaluation must include a variety of techniques and assessments, and it is also widely accepted that an authentic and natural language use is an important part of any evaluation. In an environment, however, where reports are used to qualify an individual for intervention services, secure third-party reimbursements, acquire learning accommodations, or monitor functional progress, the integrity of the authentic assessment is determined solely on the basis of the examiner's decision and ultimate reporting. There is increasing available literature on the value of authentic testing for use in assessing individuals from culturally and linguistically diverse backgrounds. This information should be carefully reviewed by evaluators as a critical component of evidence based evaluation and documentation.

THE DYNAMICS OF DYNAMIC ASSESSMENT

Dynamic assessment is one other additional type of evaluation tool that can be used by speech-language pathologists to assess aspects of language and learning to gain further information about their client's or patient's abilities. It is a form of authentic assessment in that it is not standardized, and the use and manner of a dynamic assessment will vary with the client, patient, reason for referral, and, as always, the skill and experience of the evaluator.

To briefly understand what a dynamic assessment is, consider that it analyzes an individual's ability to learn. The results can be indicative of a number of things. Tasks, skills, or areas of language that an individual may have shown weakness in during testing or in which there is reported weakness are selected and targeted by the examiner. The individual is taught the ability, task, or skill in the weakened area, and their ability to acquire the new knowledge is assessed. It is also frequently identified as an alternative type of assessment that can be used to help diagnose language ability in individuals of culturally or linguistically diverse backgrounds. It can be used as part of a differential diagnosis to identify differences from disorders. It also can help in assessing learning style, ability, and readiness. It is described as an alternative type of assessment that has specific uses in evaluation. It can provide prognostic indicators. If an evaluator chooses to include this type of assessment, as in all of their assessment tests described, they should be thoroughly familiar with its use. The evaluator should understand the concepts and techniques of dynamic assessment and when and how to best use it. Similarly understanding and appreciating the value of a dynamic assessment will lead to an understanding of how to document this aspect of the evaluation in the written diagnostic report.

In assessing a client's or patient's ability to change or learn a new task, the term "modifiability" is often used. A measurement of baseline behavior or pretest is used. An intervention that may involve prompting, cueing, teaching, modeling, or providing feedback is next used to teach the decided upon targeted task. Following the intervention, the outcome is assessed. It is an interactive type of assessment where the client's or patient's response(s) and ability to learn is evaluated.

It is up to the evaluator to decide when and for what reason to use a dynamic assessment method. It is not a standard part of every assessment and is up to the discretion of the evaluator. The dynamic type of assessment is described in many basic textbooks on evaluation and language assessment, and there are many published articles available that discuss the use of this type of assessment. Continuing education courses and even supervised administrations should be considered prior to beginning the use of dynamic assessment in evaluations if one is not familiar with its use.

DOCUMENTING THE DYNAMIC ASSESSMENT

By its very nature, a dynamic assessment is difficult to document. There is little, if anything, standardized about this type of assessment, which is one of the advantages of this technique. It allows for flexibility and creativity. It allows the evaluator to make decisions about how best to gain additional information and insight into their client or patient. The dynamic assessment opens the door to endless possibilities of areas of language to further assess, how to assess the baseline skill, what method to use to teach the skill, how to assess the client's behavior and response, and how to measure the targeted skill after teaching. The degree of subjectivity allowed in the process can understandably be immense. The dynamic process from start to finish relies on the examiner's experience, knowledge, and expertise. These same examiner qualities must then be used and transferred into the documentation portion of dynamic assessment.

In documenting the dynamic portion of the assessment, it will help the writer to remember to clearly describe the steps involved in the process. A brief explanation of what a dynamic assessment is and what the goal is may help the readers' understanding of the process. The writer then must clearly describe the steps of the dynamic assessment process as they were previously described. This of course will vary depending upon the dynamic process used determined by the evaluator's resources, references, or learning. What should be clearly documented is the selected skill that was selected to dynamically assess. If there was a specific reason for selecting this skill, why? What was the baseline ability of the skill prior to the intervention technique applied? How was it measured? If objective data were collected, specify them. How and what intervention technique was applied? Was there a specific reason the intervention was selected? If a degree or dose of intervention can be specified, that should be added and would be helpful in understanding the process. The patient's or client's responses should be indicated. This may be behavioral, clinical, quantitative, qualitative, or a combination. How was this aspect measured? Following this complicated process, there must be some discussion, perhaps in summary and recommendations, that describes what information this adds about the patient. This information can also assist in recommendations, referrals, and intervention planning, including frequency and duration of therapy sessions. This should all be integrated into the report. The skilled use of dynamic assessment, if properly applied and documented, can be a valuable addition to a client's or patient's assessment process.

REFERENCES

Bowles, R., Justice, L., Khan, K., Pista, S., Skibbe, L., & Foster, T. (2020). Development of the Narrative Assessment Protocol-2: A tool for examining young children's narrative. *Language, Speech, and Hearing Services in Schools, 51*(2), 390-404. https://doi.org/10.1044/2019_LSHSS-19-00038

Owens, R., & Pavelco, S. (2020). Sampling Utterances and Grammatical Analysis Revised (SUGAR): New normative values for language analysis measures in 8–10 year old children. *Language, Speech, and Hearing Services in Schools, 51*(3), 734-744.

Systematic Analysis of Language Transcripts. (2022). htpss://www.Saltsoftware.com

Wiig, E., Semel, E., & Secord, W. (2013). *Clinical evaluation of language fundamentals, 5th ed. (CELF-5)*. NCS Pearson.

Language Is Not Always Standard

Speech-language pathologists evaluate individuals across the life span who present with a variety of communication disorders. These can result from countless events, reasons, and etiologies. The assessment of these disorders requires specific knowledge and experience and relies on the ability to select and use a corresponding variety of assessment techniques and measures. Specific test measures have been developed and published to evaluate targeted areas and elements of communication that have been shown to be disrupted in specific diagnoses. Some of these areas include, but are not limited to, voice, resonance, reading, writing, fluency, social skills, aphasia, dementia, traumatic brain injury (TBI), and functional activities of daily living involving communication.

Documenting results of tests and measurements discussed thus far has largely emphasized standardized and norm-referenced tests for language and speech sound production areas. These areas generally rely on the use of standardized tests, especially norm referenced, that rely on straightforward scoring, familiar to most evaluators, and have numerous advantages in the ability to understand and interpret results by the majority of speech-language pathologists. The preponderance of these standardized norm-referenced tests is available for use with children, adolescents, and, in some cases, young adults. Standardized norm-referenced tests for speech sound production and language are less available for older adults. There are numerous reasons for the fact that most standardized and standardized norm-referenced assessments are made available for children and adolescents, especially in the age range of 3 to 21. Evaluators should be aware of these reasons.

Blaustein, S. H. *Diagnostic Report Writing in Speech-Language Pathology:
A Guide to Effective Communication* (pp. 79-85).
© 2023 Taylor & Francis Group.

As we evaluate older patients across the life span who present with a variety of acquired disorders such as aphasia, dementia, TBI, or postsurgical or medical conditions, function and use of the tests and measurements we rely on become more varied and less straightforward to administer and document. The nature of targeted diagnostic tests, types of scores reported, interpretation of scores, and how they should be documented in reports becomes another important area for consideration in diagnostic report writing. While many of these more varied instruments are standardized in their administration, the types of information produced, organization of each test, and scoring, analysis, and interpretation of results often may greatly vary from the typical norm-referenced reliance on comparisons to a "bell curve."

Through understanding how report writing occurs, the documentation and writing process is simplified for the evaluator who understands the basic tenets of diagnostic report writing. It is understood that the evaluator must continue to provide the full name of any standard test or measurement utilized, as well as inform the reader of the nature and purpose of the test and why it was selected. Descriptions of test components, including individual subtests and ways in which subtest scores are combined to yield core, index, total, or other defined scores, should be included. Explaining how scores are derived, analyzed, and interpreted must also be stated. Documenting examples of an individual's actual performance, including examples of correct and incorrect responses during the test, could highlight areas of strength and weakness and is helpful. Viewed in this manner, the documentation of the results and findings from these types of assessments is not difficult to report. Any novel specific reporting categories or terminology used in reporting specific scores derived, categories and considerations of how these scores are interpreted beyond the traditional standardized score model, and what the scores tell us about a client's or patient's performance must be described. The tables and charts that may be presented for some of these evaluations will also vary in their organization and terminology. They must include the relevant and important psychometric information that enables the functional use of the scores attained. As always, the accurate and documented results are necessary as part of any effective diagnostic written report. This relies on the knowledge and skills of the evaluator, including their familiarity with the test, how it is used, and why it is used. This information enables an easier incorporation of test results into the diagnostic report. Given the lack of knowledge or experience by outside readers with many tests and measurements included in our reports, any confusion in interpretation will only be exacerbated when a report is presented with imprecise and unclear test description and reporting.

An advantage of tests that utilize norm-referenced reporting is that the scores are derived from the "bell curve" that represents a normal distribution that many individuals, including parents and professionals, are familiar with. Reporting a language score in the 10th percentile clearly indicates a level of difficulty while reporting a 90th percentile score in vocabulary is an easy concept to grasp. Numerous tests that evaluate communication disorders do not provide the typical norm-referenced standard, scaled, and percentile scores that speech-language pathologists often rely on.

Many tests frequently used by speech-language pathologists do not necessarily rely on a normal distribution based on an identified population or sample with typical norm-referenced conversion tables available. Different psychometric principles, ways in which results are scored, and resulting analysis and interpretation vary in many types of tests. There are many reasons for this. Difficulty finding sufficient numbers of homogeneous groups to establish a representative sample or the type, nature, and characteristics of a specific communication disorder that might be unique and difficult to measure can create barriers to test development. Limited responsiveness of the individuals who have a particular disorder or very young or old ages can provide additional variables to how tests are developed and scored. These tests are often introduced by researchers or clinicians familiar with a particular communication disorder and who realize the need for a test to capture the critical clinical features that will be valuable in diagnosis. Many of these reasons are described in the examiner's manual, and it is necessary for the clinician to fully understand them. It may also be beneficial at times to include them in the diagnostic report to allow the reader to fully understand the test results as they relate to a client's or patient's function and diagnosis.

As with reporting standardized norm-referenced assessments, an examiner must be thoroughly familiar with the test being administered. This includes a working knowledge of the examiner's manual, including what the test is designed to measure, theoretical basis, procedures for administration, instructions on scoring, and, most importantly, how results are to be analyzed and interpreted. This information is a prerequisite to be able to document test results in the diagnostic evaluation.

An evaluator should not be intimidated or reluctant to incorporate a new test, especially one with a nontraditional or less familiar scoring methodology, into practice. In fact, speech-language pathologists should seek to remain current and evidence based and to provide the best services to the clients they serve. It is important to remain within our scope of practice and acquire the necessary knowledge and skill set to appropriately administer the test.

It is important to expand our test battery for a number of reasons. New tests are being developed and current popular tests are updated. An individual may be employed in a new work setting and called upon to evaluate a set of individuals with disorders they may not have previously encountered. Even for speech-language pathologists remaining in the same, familiar work setting, the therapist may be asked to begin doing evaluations on a different population within the setting or to assume responsibilities for a colleague that may be on leave or retire. A solo private practitioner may wish to expand a practice to include individuals of different ages or diagnoses. There are many situations in which evaluators will be called upon to administer a new "type" of test that they must eventually administer and subsequently incorporate into written diagnostic evaluation.

Looking at Other Standard Tests

Remembering that a test can be standardized but not norm referenced is an important factor in considering the use of tests. Remember that standardization of a test means specifying a manner to administer a test, specific questions, uniform stimuli, and factors put into place to ensure similar administration of the test in question. Tests, although having a standard administration protocol, may not be tied to a specific norm-referenced sample that would provide the familiar, traditional types of scores speech-language pathologists are most familiar with. Many of these tests may involve scales, questionnaires, inventories, observations, surveys, or other measures, and the analysis and use of the information gleaned from these tests may be reported in a way unique to the specific tests. There may also be assessments that rely on objective instrumentation producing data that must then be cross-referenced with available normative or descriptive published norms or descriptions. It would be impossible to provide a list and explanation of all types of tests available to speech-language pathologists that are not norm referenced. That is not the goal of this discussion but rather to increase awareness of the variability in the tests utilized by speech-language pathologists and to emphasize the continued need for clear and informed documentation.

It Is Not Always About a Norm-Referenced Score

It has already been discussed that test selection is a critical factor in the evaluation of speech and language skills. Table 9-1 includes a summary of some basic factors that go into test selection, many of which may be included in the report if they provide greater support or accountability for reported results. For the majority of preschool through college-aged students for whom we are evaluating speech, language, literacy, and related skills, most tests rely on a traditional norm-referenced scoring system. It makes sense to measure development in areas against "typical" development of skills as they are acquired by a matched peer group. The idea of development over time is important and we are able to capture the differences in this development using age-referenced sample populations. What happens when adults are in need of assessment who have already mastered adult-level communication skills? What happens when age-correlated speech and language acquisition has ceased and fully mature levels of speech, language, and related skills are present and an event has disrupted these skills?

TABLE 9-1
Factors to Consider in Test Selection
• Reason for referral
• Relevant case history information
• Available results of previous testing
• Potential diagnosis to consider or rule out
• Age of the client or patient
• Inclusion criteria for standardization sample of test
• Language and cultural variables
• Responsive level of client or patient
• Ability level of patient or client
• Barriers to testing including attention, vision, hearing, and physical limitations

Communication disorders unfortunately occur across the life span. Events such as stroke, TBI, pathologies related to medical/neurological conditions, surgeries, and dementia are a few of the events that can severely disrupt communication in an adult who has seen the attained adult level of communication skills. Evaluation of the language skills in such individuals must be determined, but the focus now will shift from academic and social developmental language to the significant loss of function that an adult may experience. This functional loss can affect work, personality, socialization, family life, and activities of daily living. Our assessments and subsequent reports may often turn primarily to the characteristics of a disorder. Evaluation of strengths and weaknesses on language tasks as they impact an individual across these functional areas becomes increasingly important. Information reported is necessary not only for diagnosis but to recommend therapeutic programs aimed at improving functional skills that will improve quality of life, work, and socialization. Accurate documentation is necessary to ensure successful placement and funding for interventions as well.

Different Disorders, Different Tests, Different Focus

It is not practical to present the many varieties of tests, measurements, and different scoring systems used to assist in diagnosing communication disorders. Reports will vary with each individual, diagnosis, reason for referral, and evaluator. Providing examples of reports or templates for each diagnosis we assess would be an admirable but impractical goal. A discussion of some broad categories of disorders where tests are commonly used that provide assessment results in manners that may not rely primarily on norm-referenced systems.

Patients presenting with neurogenic-based communication disorders vary greatly in age, specific etiology, and how the disorders manifest. Aphasia may be caused by any number of factors, including cerebrovascular accident or stroke, trauma, or infection. There are numerous standardized tests available where the primary goal is to identify or classify the type and severity of aphasia present. The tests are usually developed by authors extremely experienced and often directly involved in diagnosis, treatment, and research involving individuals diagnosed with aphasia. The tests are based on the author's understanding and theoretical framework as to how to best classify and describe the disorder, including the speech, language, reading, writing, and phonatory voice areas that can all be impacted by aphasia to varying degrees. Each modality impacted clearly disrupts an individual's quality of life. Test results describing these areas must be clearly documented based on the theoretical basis of the specified test selected and the author's specific instructions on how to score, analyze, and interpret results.

Right hemisphere dysfunction testing follows many of the same theoretical diagnostic principles as testing for aphasia. The site of lesion involves the right hemisphere and, as such, assessments are largely developed and theorized to include not only the typical areas included in aphasia diagnosis but also test items and tasks to evaluate the specific and unique characteristics of right hemisphere dysfunction. Specialized tests to assess right hemisphere dysfunction are available. Attention, perceptual deficits, problem solving, pragmatics, and prosody are areas of function targeted along with language. The condition of "neglect" is an important aspect of this disorder to note and document.

Speech-language pathologists are becoming increasingly involved in the diagnosis and interventions for individuals with communication deficits resulting from TBI. This includes coma commonly associated with a TBI diagnosis. Involvement often includes being a member of an interdisciplinary team of professionals where clear reporting, documentation, and communication are critical. Tests and measurements for TBI, as in other discrete etiologies, are available and target frequently impacted areas, including orientation, executive function, cognition, visuospatial, visuomotor, personality, and pragmatics. Speech-language pathologists should be aware of the significant types of TBI that occur and associated medical conditions, including coma. There are specific scales and measures used to assess coma and related intellectual cognitive deficits of TBI that may not be administered by the speech-language pathologist but may be necessary to include in the case history and interprofessional communications. It is therefore recommended that speech-language pathologists working in this area become familiar with the associated tests and measurement, which will not only improve diagnosis but can be better integrated into the documentation. Documenting functional baselines is extremely important for this diagnosis.

A variety of etiologies result in an associated diagnosis of dementia. Alzheimer's disease, vascular dementia, frontotemporal lobar degeneration, Lewy body dementia, Parkinson's disease, Pick's disease, and Huntington's disease are examples of the numerous and complex neurological disorders to consider. Dementia can be further conceptualized by areas of involvement such as cortical, subcortical, and mixed. The varied associated disease processes along with the concomitant medical and physical problems and progressive nature of dementia make the assessment, diagnosis, and documentation of the communication deficits a difficult process. There are numerous diagnostic features included, but they are all tied together with the establishment of memory loss as a necessary symptom to make the diagnosis of dementia. Specific tests for dementia are available and aimed at identifying the severity, areas of deficit, and impact on patient functioning. Careful documentation is called for to establish baselines of function at the specific point of assessment. The progressive nature of dementia will cause progression of symptoms from early to advanced stages with increasing and increased levels of impairment of speech, language, and related function. Levels of function become critical to placement in rehabilitation programs and documentation of progress during therapy. Precise documentation for reimbursement purposes, as always, remains important.

Neurogenic areas of communication deficit clearly impact function across the environment. Evaluators often rely on specific tests and measurements that specify a patient's functional status in day-to-day functioning. A variety of standard tests are available to assess aspects of functional communication. The American Speech-Language-Hearing Association has devoted much attention and resources to heightening awareness in the use of functional measures for its members. Functional assessments have become key for rehabilitation placements, monitoring progress, establishing intervention programs, and submitting documentation for critical insurance reimbursement. Speech-language pathologists must be aware of their use and documentation.

The American Speech-Language-Hearing Association Functional Assessment of Communication Skills for Adults is an example of a type of a standard assessment protocol that relies on a specified scoring system that needs to be correctly documented following administration (Frattali et al., 2017). It is designed to measure the functional communication skills of adults and assesses 43 items across four domains. Based on observations from the evaluator, social communication, communication of basic needs, reading/writing, number concepts, and daily living are assessed. Understanding this measure and accurately documenting results according to specified guidelines can be a valuable asset to an evaluator's assessment repertoire.

Neurogenic etiologies also impact children and adolescents. Similar careful attention must be paid to selection of test instruments with careful attention given to how these tests are administered, used, and reported. Any alterations, adaptations, or modifications to test administration that vary from the examiner's manual guidelines must be noted in the report. Scores provided in standard tests are based on administration of stimuli as directed, and changes in how tests are administered, although often needed, impact the reliability of scores provided. Providing repetitions of a prompt when none are allowed or providing additional auditory cues beyond the prompts provided are examples of changes that should be reported. Given the age level of children and adolescent patients, there are numerous standardized, norm-referenced language tests available. When using any standardized norm-referenced test for children and adolescents with acquired communication disorders, even if they fall within the age limits of the test, it is extremely important to realize that these disorders are acquired and not developmental. Attention must be given to psychometric test standardization principles, including the standardization populations, inclusion of children and adolescents with acquired communication disorders in standardization samples, and any changes made to the manner of test administration. Any variations should be noted and test scores may not be allowed to be reported. Resulting scores can be misleading and incorrect. Descriptions of performance can be described and results should be noted to be "for descriptive" or "for comparative" purposes.

Beyond acquired neuropathies in children and adolescents, there are other disorders where specific types of assessments are used that report results unique to the disorder with scoring developed specifically for those unique elements. Standard tests for fluency, although containing norm-referenced scoring, often involve other relevant measures specific to the disorder, including information on percentages of stuttered words, length of prolongations, descriptions of secondary behaviors, or other types of dysfluencies. Tests are also available that are used to assess perceptions, feelings, and attitudes of individuals who stutter with reporting metrics that may use rating scales or other measures that must be clearly explained in the final written report.

Numerous rating scales are available to speech-language pathologists to assist in the assessment and diagnosis of autism spectrum disorders (ASDs). Again, evaluators often rely on the many standardized norm-referenced assessments available in the 3- to 21-year age level but must be aware of limitations in administering tests and reporting results based on the information provided in each examiner's manual. Language and behavior scales, based on similar observations used in the *Diagnostic and Statistical Manual of Mental Disorders, Fifth Edition* (American Psychiatric Association, 2013) for diagnosing ASDs, including evaluator ratings and caregiver interviews, assess areas that are considered in the diagnosis and severity of ASD. Clear documentation and explanation of these tests, how scores are developed and gathered, and what results mean should be provided in the written diagnostic evaluation.

Another type of evaluation where reported results are standardized, where test scoring is variable and more individualized to each test instrument, is in assessment of infants and toddlers. There are rating scales, questionnaires, parent interviews, inventories, observations, and other types of tests available to assess communication and related skills from birth through 3. Unique scoring systems are available and must be included along with their explanations when documenting. One such example is the MacArthur-Bates Communicative Development Inventories–Second Edition (Fenson & Marchman, 2007), which assesses early language development in 8- to 30-month-old children. It is based on caregiver questionnaires and results are largely presented in percentile scores rather than scaled or standard scores. This assessment is frequently used in research, has been translated into many languages, and has diagnostic clinical value. To illustrate the different and unique ways in which test scores may be reported, the test developers state,

"Percentile scores are not appropriate for some sections" (Fenson & Marchman, 2007, pp. 29-30). They then indicate the Words and Gestures segment of the test where two specific measurements, "First Signs of Understanding" and "Starting to Talk," do not rely on percentile scores to report. Clinicians are directed to "additional specific instructions" for interpretation of these sections. Reporting and documentation must reflect these interpretations of results.

Communication disorders assessed by speech-language pathologists are numerous and varied. They range from infants to older adults and from ASD to dementia. The numbers and types of tests and measures available are as diverse as the disorders we evaluate. The manner in which these tests are administered, scored, and analyzed further reflects this diversity. The speech-language pathologist must be proficient in correctly, professionally, and functionally documenting and explaining the instruments that are used in our testing. We must be confident that our reports are reliable and functional and have value to our clients and patients for whatever reason the report is generated.

References

American Psychiatric Association. (2013). *Diagnostic and statistical manual of mental disorders* (5th ed.).

Fenson, L., & Marchman, V. (2007). *Macarthur-Bates communicative development inventories* (2nd ed.). Brookes.

Frattali, C. M., Thompson, C. K., Holland, A. L., Wohl, C. B., Wenck, C. J., Slater, S. C., & Paul, D. (2017). *American Speech-Language-Hearing Association Functional Assessment of Communication Skills for Adults (ASHA FACS)*. ASHA.

You Need to Know More
Specific Documentation by Setting

Speech-language pathologists spend a great deal of time during their training learning the necessary knowledge and skills to perform diagnostic evaluations. A diagnostic speech and language evaluation report must then be completed to share the results of that evaluation with others. Unfortunately, due to large numbers of students, additional required clinical hours and responsibilities, coursework, and externships and other requirements, many students will earn their degrees with only limited diagnostic and report writing experiences. There is a great deal to learn, including obtaining and utilizing case history information; how to select, use, and score tests; and eventually how to use the information gathered to determine a diagnosis. Specific recommendations and referrals must also be decided upon and included. Consider that the diagnostic process must be learned and practiced in a variety of courses that may include child and adult language disorders, voice disorders, fluency disorders, aphasia, dysphagia, and autism. Students must also learn and practice all of the associated knowledge and skills that accompany these evaluations. Part of the process includes professional report writing and how to best share information with clients, patients, families, and other professionals. While most clinical courses will include basic information about assessment in the curriculum such as the names of tests and symptoms of disorders, this theoretical base often lacks associated face-to-face practical experience with actual clients and patients experiencing the variety of disorders that are studied theoretically. The limited experience in writing diagnostic reports becomes an unfortunate but understandable aspect of graduate education. It is true that

Blaustein, S. H. *Diagnostic Report Writing in Speech–Language Pathology: A Guide to Effective Communication* (pp. 87-97).
© 2023 Taylor & Francis Group.

the recent pandemic has allowed more clinical hours through simulated cases and more exposure through telepractice, but for students, there is no substitute for actual face-to-face clinical contact. Assessing remotely is a very different experience than completing an in-person evaluation.

Given the time and practical constraints in graduate school education, it is unlikely that a student will have had the opportunity to complete but a few supervised clinical evaluations from initial intake to final written report. There certainly will not be the opportunity to complete evaluations across a wide variety of disorders and settings. Much of the needed information to complete assessments and evaluations in speech-language pathology is learned theoretically in the numerous required courses and electives that students complete. Learning information theoretically does not necessarily mean acquiring the actual clinical competencies to complete the required diagnostic tasks. Too often, students understand theoretical concepts, can memorize the names of tests, and can state symptoms that underlie the diagnosis. These same students often struggle when it comes to applying these skills in actual clinical practice where the evaluation must be completed, analyzed, and results documented. That is the reason many programs are switching to competency-based assessments of students' performance in addition to solely assessing students' theoretical knowledge. They do not necessarily go hand in hand.

Given the limitations on report writing learning opportunities, it stands to reason that programs struggle to devise and offer the best possible experiences to teach students to be basic competent diagnosticians and report writers. Hours are spent following the completion of the diagnostic evaluations with students handing in drafts, often multiple times, to be reviewed and edited by their clinical supervisors. The process can be time-consuming and laborious. It may be one of the reasons students may not appreciate and learn to develop a passion for the diagnostic process. Priorities taught involve developing a basic skill set of assessing, administering a limited number of tests, diagnosing, and documenting evaluations. These are the primary and most important aspects of an evaluation and must be done at the highest level of basic competency. There are, however, other aspects and skills that must be considered and included in an evaluation that serves other needs for our assessments. These may sometimes be more clearly obvious, understood, and stated, yet in other instances, they may be more subtle or implied but must be clearly understood and considered by the evaluator. These additional functions an evaluation serves may be just read about or briefly touched on in graduate school training and are often not highlighted during training as an important part of the evaluation process. Students may be so focused on mastering the basic skills of assessment and writing that the more nuanced and subtle aspects do not seem important. It is often during a student's Clinical Fellowship (CF) that more specific and secondary goals to be included in a report are specified. These are specific to a setting, such as a school or skilled nursing facility, and are taught or presented in templates to be used, but again, this skill set is often later acquired dependent on an individual's CF placement, supervisor, and requirements within a unique situation.

The careful assessment, diagnosis, recommendation, and referrals for an individual client or patient undeniably complete a critical first step in a process. The successful evaluation is only the culmination of one step in the process. It is in the next phase of the process, writing the diagnostic report, where the value of the assessment will be functionally proven. It is in providing the conclusions, impressions, recommendations, and referrals where the secondary underlying goals of an evaluation play a critical role, a role that in many cases becomes essential in determining the outcome for the patient. This is as important as completing the initial evaluation. As successful as a diagnostic evaluation may be in carefully and adequately assessing a patient by providing a diagnosis and recommendations, it is less useful if required information in that report is lacking. It will prevent the patient from continuing with the rehabilitation and intervention process. Outcomes require documentation that supports the desired outcome selected by the evaluator, family, and other parties involved, including physicians.

Multiple Goals for an Evaluation: Know What Is Needed

The specific documentation for various disorders that is required to attain placement, funding, or services is detailed in a variety of documents that literally generate hundreds and hundreds of pages. Documentation requirements are contained in numerous documents available to clinicians, and evaluators should be aware of their existence and where to find them. The disorders and treatments assessed, diagnosed, and treated range from communication deficits associated with autism spectrum disorders to dementia associated with Alzheimer's disease to laryngectomy and stuttering. Statutes, laws, insurance policy manuals, requirements, and regulations specify what an individual must currently demonstrate, may have previously had, does not have, or what diagnostic grouping they must be part of to attain what is needed in the next phase of a rehabilitation journey. Numerous agencies, government entities, educational institutions, and insurance companies, to name a few examples, all generate specific written guidelines specifying information that must be documented in a report to allow approval or denial of services. Without meeting specified conditions, without clearly documenting and supporting these findings, and without clearly stating results, descriptions, and outcomes that are desired by a requesting body, any number of essential services, including funding, will easily be denied. In many cases, the diagnosis becomes just the first part of a long road for the patient. It is unfortunate when a patient meets the criteria for inclusion in a program, setting, or funding opportunity and is then denied approval because of insufficient documentation or knowledge.

It is not practical to include all of the many complex and detailed specifics of the numerous guidelines, regulations, and rules that specify the unique criteria that must be included in reports to ensure services. In fact, it is impossible. Suffice it to say that an evaluator must be aware that these guidelines exist, are specific to individual clients or patients, are related to various recommendations and referrals for a variety of disorders, and must be recognized and clearly incorporated into written diagnostic evaluations where appropriate. The evaluator should know where to find this information and when it should be used.

Speech-language pathologists are employed in a variety of employment settings. Requirements for a specific style of documentation will vary by the specific work environment. There usually will be a broad template provided by employers to ensure consistency among clinicians and to reduce wide variations in reports that all bear the name of a specific setting. The final content and style of any report will depend on numerous factors, including the age of the client, the specific setting of the evaluation, reason for referral, tests administered, and diagnosis. Recommendations for intervention and referrals to other professionals if needed are also generally part of completed reports.

Speech-language pathologists learning to conduct evaluations are aware that primary goals of an evaluation are to assess an individual for a possible communication disorder, consider presence or absence of the disorder, diagnose, and make recommendations. Successful clinicians will demonstrate competence in these areas prior to employment and improve these skills with experience and time.

Secondary Evaluation Goals

What many clinicians do not realize early in their educational careers is that evaluations, as complex as they are, often have important secondary goals. What is meant by a "secondary goal" of an evaluation? Specifying a diagnosis, recommendation, and referrals is often just the beginning of a process for a client or patient. What follows may be weeks, months, or even years of interventions. Outpatient or inpatient, placements may need to be approved and students may need to qualify for a variety of services provided by school districts. Third-party payers, including Medicare, Medicaid, and private pay insurance companies, may need to authorize reimbursements for many necessary interventions and programs. Each of these situations will require careful review of the speech and language evaluation. Just because an individual has been evaluated and receives a diagnosis and a recommendation for therapy does not automatically guarantee that placements, interventions, or funding will be approved. Reviewers and auditors seek very specific information within a report that will allow them to approve or qualify a client, patient, or student for a desired outcome. Clearly providing this necessary information for the reader will facilitate a desired outcome.

Two examples of broad categories where very specific requirements must be met will be detailed. Each of the examples provided will illustrate specific situations where information to be provided within the evaluation report must clearly meet any criteria set forth by the party, which must review the report and certify that all of the guidelines have been met to approve the request of the client or patient. This "secondary goal" must be acknowledged by the clinician, demonstrated by inclusion into the written documentation. The evaluator must be aware of the requisite information to be included that meets the ultimate goals of the client, patient, and others involved in the care of the individual being evaluated.

While the primary goal of an assessment is to evaluate the client or patient, determine the existence and severity of a disorder, and make recommendations, there are other factors to be considered beyond the diagnosis and recommendations. The secondary goal is therefore to be aware of the specific documentation requirements needed for those outcomes to be successful. That means the evaluator must be keenly aware of the exact wording, content, and inclusion or exclusion requirements to gain approval for a desired outcome.

It is essential to state here that this must be honestly provided, well supported, and clear. There are times when a client or patient may ask for a different diagnosis, exaggeration of symptoms, or increase in recommendations provided. As innocent as this may seem, it is never to be done. It is a violation of our Code of Ethics and can jeopardize our state licensure, and it is unethical, if not illegal, to document information that is not entirely factual. In our desire to assist a family we have worked with to be approved for a service or placement, providing misleading information can have severe consequences for the evaluator. The integrity and reputation of every evaluator must remain the highest priority. The eventual desired outcome may be approval of recommendations for provision of services, placement at a desired setting, funding, or a combination of many of these. This is done via comprehensive evaluation and documentation.

The two specific sets of requirements presented highlight the complexities of required documentation by setting and the variation in the skill and knowledge set necessary. The requirements for Early Intervention, which covers birth to 3 years (through 2 years 11 months), and requirements for individuals in inpatient rehabilitation facilities (IRFs) as funded by Medicare for individuals age 65 and older will be highlighted with respect to their unique requirements.

The diagnostic requirements of each setting will be described in addition to the layers of regulations that necessitate specific information in a report, where the requirements for this information originate, the regulatory agencies involved, and the speech-language pathologist's role and responsibilities within the setting. To emphasize the range of clients, patients, and disorders that speech-language pathologists assess and provide treatment for, two examples at opposite ends of the life span are discussed.

Inpatient Rehabilitation Facility Requirements

Speech-language pathologists are employed by or provide consulting and contract services to IRFs. These specialized medical settings serve as discharge options for hospital-based patients who are in need of specialized rehabilitation and skilled medical care. As part of hospital-based discharge planning, an interprofessional team, familiar with the patient's diagnosis, hospital course, and needs, may decide that an IRF is the best option upon discharge for a patient under review.

In order for this referral to be successful, transfer of the patient and funding for the setting must be approved. A very clear set of requirements must be met and the referring setting must ensure that the patient is appropriate for the setting prior to making the recommendation to the patient and family. The documentation of these requirements becomes a critical factor. In fact, it is so critical that if one were to visit the Centers for Medicare & Medicaid Services (CMS) website (CMS, n.d.), among the detailed information provided is a list of common inpatient rehabilitation therapy service errors. These "errors" refer to errors in documentation within these settings, and they ultimately may result in lack of approval for the requested placement, reimbursement, and/or provision of services. It is useful to view the errors provided by CMS as they occur so frequently that they are indicated for providers on the CMS website.

The first error listed is **"documentation does not support medical necessity."** The medical necessity determination is critical to determination of approvals, and it further states that **"admission is reasonable and necessary based on assessment of individual's needs at time of admission."** Prior to understanding the requirements that are necessary for speech-language pathologists involved in making referrals to and working with patients in inpatient rehabilitation settings, it is important to note how critical documentation is within this setting. One must understand what information the individuals who review patients' medical records who are applying for or placed within these settings are looking for. Including the required information in documentation and presenting it in a clear manner that reviewers can easily recognize is important. Knowing what information is required and determining that your patient meets necessary criteria for approval is critical. This becomes a secondary goal of the report that will accompany the information that will be provided to the accepting facility. All criteria should therefore be understood by the speech pathologist assessing and documenting a patient's needs within inpatient rehabilitation. This will undoubtedly be part of any clinician's orientation by the facility prior to employment. A clinician demonstrating this knowledge prior to employment will certainly be an advantage for those seeking work in such a setting.

Criteria for inpatient rehabilitation specify that active and ongoing intervention from multiple disciplines is a requirement for placement, and speech-language pathology is one of the approved disciplines that may be an intervention. It is further stated that physical therapy and/or occupational therapy must be one of the provided specified multidisciplinary interventions and that the patient requires intensive rehabilitation. Other factors to consider in documentation of patients within inpatient rehabilitation settings is that the patient is expected to be able to actively participate in their therapies, and it is essential that the patient also be able to benefit significantly from their interventions. A speech-language pathologist, as part of the hospital-based discharge team or IRF rehabilitation team, must be aware of these criteria and be sure that information supporting the requirements is included in their reports.

The CMS requirements are very specific in identifying and defining required elements of an evaluation, and it must be assumed that these elements will be reviewed and assessed through a review prior to placement for approval and payment. One such requirement is that a patient's functional status be stated. It is further stated that the patient is expected to make **"measurable improvement."** These factors are written in a very straightforward manner and are stated in CMS regulations and have clear implications. Functional status on admission and throughout therapy presents a need to describe from a communication and swallowing point of view specifically what skills the patient is able to functionally display. Additionally, it must be specified that there is a prognosis for expected improvement and that this improvement has to be documented in a measurable way. Thus, initial assessments must make this clear in ways that can be "measured." The clinician must use standard tests and authentic measures that will provide measurements that relate to these requirements. Absent this documentation in an evaluation, approval can be jeopardized. Progress in communication skills through ongoing assessments must relate to initial measures determined and goals specified. Continued placement in an IRF is dependent upon ongoing assessment of the intensive multidisciplinary rehabilitation that a patient is receiving and the certification of an interdisciplinary approach where the patient, in a measured way, is functionally improving. There are other specific terms, including that the improvement should be ongoing, sustainable, and of practical value. Reports must be prepared in a manner that recognizes and uses the required terminology. These are factors that may not necessarily be needed in reports written for patients presenting with other communication disorders.

It is essential that speech-language pathologists working within IRF settings thoroughly understand the requirements. It is clear that they are based on assessments and evaluation where a diagnosis has already been made. It is relevant that any initial evaluation reports and subsequent assessments must refer to the initial assessment, the functional goals, and the degree of progress. This must be specified in a way that is easily identifiable and recognizable to reviewers of medical records for the IRFs.

Further review of documentation requirements within an IRF includes specifications for pre-admission screenings and **"comprehensive evaluation of condition and need for rehabilitation"** (CMS, 2021). One can further refer to the American Speech-Language-Hearing Association (ASHA) website (ASHA, n.d.) and, within their professional practice management area, specifically find information on "documentation of skilled vs. unskilled care for Medicare beneficiaries." ASHA reviews many of the elements previously discussed referring to the fact that all services must be medically necessary but adds information important not only for speech-language pathologists but all therapists working within an IRF setting. ASHA guidelines (ASHA, 2008) remind speech-language pathologists that the provision of services is of a nature that the **"level of complexity and sophistication of intervention requires a speech-language pathologist."** The complexity and sophistication aspect of the speech-language pathologist provider provision includes that there be expertise, knowledge, clinical judgment, and decision making involved that specifically require a trained and properly licensed and certified speech-language pathologist. It goes on to state that the level of care must be such that assistants, qualified personnel, and caretakers for the patient cannot provide these services independently (Medicare Benefit Policy Manual, Chapter 15, Section 220.3b).

ASHA, in providing guidelines for speech-language pathologists working within IRF settings, provides examples of what should be documented as **"skilled"** services (ASHA, 2008). These services include analyzing medical/behavioral data, selecting appropriate evaluation tools/protocols to determine communication/swallowing diagnosis and prognosis, establishing long- and short-term measurable functional goals with discharge criteria, and being able to modify activities based on expert observation. Again, ongoing assessment of patient response is another critical element (220.2c and d).

Further review of the information provided by ASHA includes points that have been discussed elsewhere in this book: that the reports, documentation, and evaluations to be reviewed by Medicare will be reviewed by professionals other than speech-language pathologists. It is stated that much of this review is conducted by Medicare-contracted nurses. As such, it is highlighted that one should not assume that the individual reading the reports will understand why a speech-language pathologist, as a skilled professional, is necessary to provide the services indicated. It is suggested that additional information be provided to clarify the necessity for the skilled service. Not only must the functional status, treatment recommendations, measurable functional goals, and outcomes be clearly reported in terms familiar to the speech-language pathologist that within our professional language clearly indicates the conditions and needs, but additional descriptors must also be put in place to enable a reviewer to easily determine the information and the justifications and meanings of the information provided. The discussion on IRF services ends with the important point that therapy services are only payable if information provided for review "consistently and accurately reports the coverage services." This important notation is critical for speech-language pathologists to understand. Documentation within any setting, whether it be a school, hospital, or IRF, not only describes an individual's status, diagnosis, recommendations, and referrals but is significant in decisions of placement and reimbursement. Denied reimbursements in an IRF due to poor documentation, lack of information, or omitted critical elements will result in denial of payment for significant reimbursements that are necessary for facilities to function and remain open. Initial denials of claims, often accompanied by requests for additional documentation, assuming the documentation is present and can be provided, result in additional paperwork, essential time that can be more efficiently spent in other activities, possible influences on a speech-language pathologist's work performance reviews, and disruptions in patient care. If the information is not available, has not been documented, or is not retrievable, the result will be eventual denial of services, loss of time, denied payment, and retrieval of payments already made. The importance of understanding necessary aspects of documentation beyond a basic speech and language evaluation within every varied medical setting cannot be understated.

ASSESSMENTS THROUGH EARLY INTERVENTION: SAME IDEA, DIFFERENT CONTENT

To provide a different set of requirements that will demonstrate the unique documentation requirements by setting, we turn to a discussion of required documentation for Early Intervention. This will serve in contrast to the detailed IRF requirements previously discussed. The basic constructs presented regarding the importance of reports having to contain not only the results of a comprehensive evaluation but having to also meet the guidelines specified by requesting parties will be evident. The idea of the "secondary goal" continues to apply.

Two speech-language pathologists may have graduated from the same program at the same time. Both will have been exposed to similar graduate-level evaluation and report writing experiences with some variation by the diagnostic cases assigned or externship placements. When employed, the reports that will need to be generated in a possible CF experience will suddenly vary greatly based on the specific site. There is no guarantee that students will have had the necessary diagnostic assessment and documentation experience to match their eventual employment setting as there is no guarantee of where a student will be employed when they graduate. Having a basic understanding of how reports are generated and being able to quickly learn and understand a setting's documentation requirements are valuable skills. Reviewing another broad and recognized program's requirements, Early Intervention, will further illustrate variations in setting requirements and provide an additional example of how there is always more that one needs to know in writing speech and language evaluations. Understanding that each diagnostic evaluation conceptually will contain similar processes and form that is then modified to include specific elements required by a referral source should make the entire process more manageable. It will serve as a guide to complete the report writing puzzle that may exist.

UNDERSTANDING EARLY INTERVENTION

Early Intervention programs (EIPs) throughout the United States employ speech-language pathologists to assess, evaluate, and provide interventions to thousands of children from birth through 2 years 11 months. Early Intervention is a program designed to improve outcomes for children with a variety of disabilities from birth through 21 years of age. This program, under the Individuals with Disabilities Education Act (IDEA) and administered by the Office of Special Education Programs, provides grants for states to provide service programs for infants and young children and their families. Under the IDEA, this program is specified in Part C.

These programs and their regulations, readily available on the U.S. Department of Education website (Early Childhood Technical Assistance Center, 2012–2020), provide specific information about the program. Under Section 1431, IDEA states that there is "a need to enhance development during a child's first 3 years of life (birth to 3)." The regulation goes on to specify a policy where financial assistance is provided to the states that will establish and provide Early Intervention services for infants and toddlers.

Under Section 1435, IDEA further discusses that provision will be through statewide systems, and the states will define the terms for developmental delay "in order to appropriately identify infants and toddlers with disabilities in need of services." The IDEA and its provision for Early Intervention broadly lays out a plan with specific requirements that will be interpreted and carried out on a state-by-state basis. Among those requirements is a "timely and comprehensive multidisciplinary evaluation of function." Speech-language pathologists play an important role in multidisciplinary evaluation.

It is not practical to specify all of the regulations and requirements for each state. As the EIP enables states to take the lead in establishing specific criteria for young children within their state, the specific requirements, regulations, and provisions are extensive. To illustrate what a specific state's system looks like, a discussion of the requirements in the State of New York will follow.

It is incumbent on each speech-language pathologist who chooses to work within Early Intervention to become aware of the regulations for the state within which they practice. Requirements, specific assessments, and documentation are specific to each state's program and will eventually result in the decisions being made as to whether a child will or will not "qualify" for an EIP and receive services asked for. In addition to the speech-language pathologist being aware of a state's basic assessment and diagnosis requirements, it becomes more critical to understand how to document and clearly show the results. Failure to understand the necessary documentation within a service provision system will certainly result in denial of services based on lack of necessary documentation.

The New York State Department of Health website (2021), with the Department of Health being responsible for mediating service positions under Early Intervention, provides a review of Early Intervention guidelines as specified in the IDEA. The user is reminded that "states have significant responsibility for defining eligibility requirements." The New York State Department of Health (2002) further goes on to specify that states define "the developmental areas, procedures, including clinical opinion, that will lead to the measure of a child's development of function." The state's criteria will decide what constitutes a developmental delay. The role of the state is further reiterated in again reminding the public that the state also defines the criteria and procedures to determine "conditions that have a high probability of resulting in a developmental delay." The speech-language pathologist can then see the role of the federal government in establishing a broad program for provision of services to find and identify young children with developmental delays and disorders, including those of communication and hearing, and how that role is then passed on to the state. Individual states then hold responsibility for creating guidelines for identification, assessment, and inclusion criteria within the individual state. The speech pathologist working in such a setting must understand the overall concepts and spirit of the EIP and further understand the clinician's role in meeting the criteria as specified. This will vary from state to state. This is what must be clearly evident in a speech and language evaluation that will be reviewed to determine eligibility for services.

What an Early Intervention Evaluator Needs to Know

Having established that each state designs specific criteria, we can continue to see what this will look like in a specific state, New York. It is clarified under EIP regulation 10 NYCRR 69.4.1(g) that assessments should be "measured by qualified personnel using '**informed clinical opinion, appropriate diagnostic procedures and/or instruments and documented for eligibility purposes.**'" Relevant for speech-language pathologists, we note the specification of "qualified" personnel, meaning duly state-licensed and certified speech-language pathologists, and the specific mention of "appropriate diagnostic procedures, clinical opinion and documentation." It is further specified that this must be done for eligibility purposes, meaning the determination of whether a child under the program will qualify for the services requested. Note that Early Intervention further specifies that "informed clinical opinion" may be used as part of the assessment. The clinician is permitted here to use their own knowledge and experience to support the findings of the evaluation. In providing clinical opinions, the evaluator is encouraged here by the author to consider evidence-based practice, and a review of the constructs contained always proves helpful in all aspects of clinical practice. The evaluator should also be aware that New York State provides "guidelines" that the clinician may use to help in providing their informed clinical opinion. New York State provides a separate appendix in their rules and regulations that lists indicators for likelihood of continued communication delay, and the speech-language pathologist must be aware of these indicators and be sure to clearly document they are present and provide specific support information based on their experience, training, and clinical judgment.

For the speech-language pathologist completing the evaluation, what is not specifically stated and inherent in this regulation is specifically what appropriate "diagnostic procedures and instruments" that must be selected consist of. The selected standardized measures vary by case and clinician. Reading numerous Early Intervention reports reveals the numerous tests, measures, scales, and questionnaires that can be used. The documentation for eligibility is also specified, that is, what results must be clearly indicated that will allow the Early Intervention program to approve intervention services for the child evaluated.

Specific criteria are provided that will enable a child to "qualify" for inclusion into the EIP and therefore receive services funded through the program. The following criteria are noted for the New York State program.

- 12-month delay in one or more functional areas
- 33% delay in one area or 25% in two areas
- If standardized instruments are used, 2 standard deviations below the mean in one area or 1.5 standard deviations below the mean in two areas

Thus, the speech-language pathologist working through Early Intervention must be aware of the appropriate assessment procedures to use and have them clearly documented.

In reviewing the criteria provided by the program, it is clear what must be documented in order for a child to be eligible for services. What is less specific is how the determination of the delay is to be quantified and what is meant by "functional areas." In understanding functional areas, these include communication, swallowing, physical therapy, and occupational therapy. A 12-month delay is easy to interpret. A 35-month-old child must be functioning at the level of a 23-month-old child (12-month delay) to qualify. Again, what is less clear is exactly how this 12-month delay will be specified, but the procedures must be determined by the speech-language pathologist and the results must be clearly documented so that a reviewer will be able to make the determination. Similarly, a 25% delay, which would be approximately 27 months, would suffice, but only if there is a 25% delay in another designated area of function. The obvious question here is the way the evaluator will document these percentages of function.

The regulation continues that if one is using standardized assessment instruments, then (scores) 2 standard deviations below the mean in one area or 1.5 standard deviations below the mean in two areas must be demonstrated. Again, it is incumbent upon the evaluator to clearly choose the appropriate test and provide the results in such a way that a reviewer is able to determine that the child meets the criteria.

There is a lot of information to be aware of in assessing a child for Early Intervention that goes well beyond simply writing a report. Understanding the eligibility requirements will enable the clinician to be sure to include all the necessary elements; present them in a well-supported, specific way addressing each eligibility requirement as described; and summarize the need for services, possible diagnosis, if present, and relevant supports. Should services be denied for some reason, which happens, clearly specifying the information in the report will be extremely useful to the speech-language pathologist in any mediation or appeal. If this information is absent, it is difficult to later say it was there, it was not included, or not enough information was provided.

The speech-language pathologist must also be aware that eligibility requirements specify that "no single measure may be used," which is a usual requirement in many education assessments to determine eligibility, including Committee on Preschool Special Education (CPSE) and Committee on Special Education. It is further required that if a standardized test is used, it should be done in combination with other procedures that include observations, teacher reports, diagnostic tests, and record reviews. It is again emphasized that an evaluator's test scores must be used in combination with multiple sources of information. An evaluator unaware of these regulations who uses a single test as the only criterion, even if the child scores specifically below the 2 standard deviations required on a test or using a qualitative measure of a 33% delay, might be denied eligibility based on failing to meet the criteria of multiple measures for assessment. It is the responsibility of the evaluator to be aware of all of these specific criteria that must be met to best document results, clearly specify them in a diagnostic evaluation, and present them in such a manner that any reviewer or committee has no question that the criteria are present and satisfied. As previously discussed, an evaluator may also use "a preponderance of specified clinical clues or indicators" if the specified criteria are not specifically met. The evaluator must further be aware of what the specified clues and indicators are, demonstrate a "preponderance," and be certain they are included along with the additional information required to best advocate for eligibility and services for the child they are evaluating.

YOU NEED TO KNOW MORE

The two programs discussed, IRF and Early Intervention, serve to demonstrate that when it comes to providing diagnostic evaluations and diagnostic reports, speech-language pathologists more than likely will need to know more about diagnostic report writing than they were prepared for. This will also be the case if one were to change work settings. The key is to know this, not be surprised by this, and expect it. Knowing how to write a basic evaluation, understanding the logic of the basic components, and being prepared to learn some new knowledge and skills will simplify the process. There is no need to be overwhelmed but rather embrace the experience as the next step in one's career path.

One has to be aware of many unique and specific documentation regulations that each work setting requires to meet the requisites for placement, provision of services, and, perhaps ultimately, and importantly, reimbursement for those services. The requirements for documentation within each of these settings are varied, broad, and clearly specified by federal, state, and local agencies; government entities; and third-party payers. It would be impossible to specify the documentation requirements for assessments for each of the work settings within which speech pathologists are employed. These numerous and unique requirements need to be clearly specified in our speech and language evaluations and made apparent in diagnostic report writing. They are learned as part of each clinician's unique employment skill set specific to unique settings.

REFERENCES

American Speech-Language-Hearing Association. (n.d.). *Documentation of skilled vs. unskilled care for Medicare beneficiaries.* https://www.asha.org/Practice/reimbursement//medicare/documentation-of-skilled-vs.-unskilled-care-for Medicare-beneficiaries/policy/KS2008-00292/

American Speech-Language-Hearing Association. (2008). *Core language and skills in speech-language pathology practice.* https://www.asha.org/

Centers for Medicare & Medicaid Services. (n.d.). *Inpatient rehabilitation therapy services: Complying with documentation requirements.* https://www.cms.gov/outreach-and-education/medicare-learning-network-mln/mlnproducts/downloads/inpatient_rehab_fact_sheet_icn905643.pdf

Early Childhood Technical Assistance Center. (2012–2020). *Part C of IDEA.* https://ectacenter.org/partc/partc.asp

New York State Department of Health. (2002). *Early Intervention: Report of the recommendations-communication disorders.* https://www.health.ny.gov/community/infants_children/early_intervention/disorders/

New York State Department of Health. (2021). *Early Intervention program.* https://www.health.ny.gov/community/infants_children/early_intervention/

BIBLIOGRAPHY

American Speech-Language-Hearing Association. (2008). *Roles and responsibilities of speech language pathologists in Early Intervention: Position statement.* https://www.asha.org/policy/ps2008–00291/

Centers for Medicare & Medicaid Services. (2016). *Medicare benefit policy manual services under hospital insurance.* https://www.cms.gov/Regulations-and-Guidance/Guidance/Manuals/downloads/bp102c01.pdf

Centers for Medicare & Medicaid Services. (2017). *Therapy services. LCD—Speech-Language Pathology (SLP) Services: Communication Disorders (L35070).* https://www.cms.gov

Centers for Medicare & Medicaid Services. (2021). *Medicare benefit policy manual-functional reporting.* https://www. https://www.cms.gov/Regulations-and-Guidance/Guidance/Manuals/Downloads/bp102c15.pdf#page=195

U.S. Department of Education. (2018). *IDEA; Part 303 (Part C). Early Intervention Program for Infants and Toddlers with Disabilities.* https://sites.ed.gov/idea/regs/c

Summary and Impressions
Time to Put It All Together

Documenting and creating the summary and impressions section of a speech and language evaluation is perhaps the most critical goal of the entire diagnostic report. It demands the greatest degree of analytical and critical thinking by the clinician and demands the entirety of one's knowledge, skills, intuition, insight, and experience. The evaluator must consider all of the objective and subjective data collected during the assessment and integrate, synthesize, and fuse all of the results to determine a hypothesis that will yield a diagnostic impression. This is where the astute clinician will present all of the collected evidence to make a case for a well-supported and documented conclusion. The conclusion, or diagnostic impression, if correctly documented and supported will enable the reader to more easily understand the communication disorder of the individual being evaluated. It will also make it easier for readers to approve whatever services, placement, or funding is being requested. Evidence-based decision making, a core element of our profession, uses the word "evidence" for a reason. Evidence is the facts that determine whether an idea, theory, statement, or proposition is valid. In our summary and impressions section, we must clearly present evidence that the conclusions we are drawing are true. To produce a fair and balanced report, it is also important for the evaluation to include and specify areas of relative strength and ability that were demonstrated throughout the assessment.

Blaustein, S. H. *Diagnostic Report Writing in Speech–Language Pathology: A Guide to Effective Communication* (pp. 99-105).

THE IMPORTANCE OF THE SUMMARY AND IMPRESSIONS

The reason that the initial referral was made, salient information from the case history, and all of the results collected from the standardized and authentic tests, observations, and measurements and assessments used throughout the evaluation must be considered as a whole. Remember that the information included, as in every section of the diagnostic report, is at the discretion and judgment of the clinician. The process involves putting together the pieces of the diagnostic puzzle and then analyzing and integrating the results. The most relevant, important, and significant information must be distinguished from the less important, confounding, and ultimately inconsequential data collected. The important parts must then be synthesized to create a hypothesis. This hypothesis will, in fact, become a working diagnosis. The ultimate goal of a speech and language evaluation is to identify and recognize a disorder or establish a reason that best explains the communication difficulty expressed by the client, answers the question concerning the reason for the referral, and explains underlying disruptions in communication processes. The diagnosis will ultimately lead to recommendations, determinations of interventions, prognosis, and possible additional referrals. This diagnosis will become the "label" for the disorder that will be used for numerous purposes, including classifications in educational settings, reimbursements, placements, and discharge planning. This information will also be used to put in place an array of modifications, adaptations, and environmental supports in school, employment, and home settings. The summary and impressions section is the clinician's opportunity to document their findings and conclusions in a cohesive and well-integrated manner for the reader. It will be the last thing read before considering the clinician's recommendations, so it must be convincing. Providing the summary and clinician's impression is the final goal of a successful evaluation. This is solely determined by the evaluator and will bear the evaluator's signature and credentials at the end of the report. It is the evaluator who will be responsible for the information contained in the report, be accountable for the diagnosis, and at some point may be called upon to defend the work presented. This may be a hearing, mediation, appeal, or possible legal case.

The information presented in the summary and impressions section is used in responses and appeals to insurance companies, read by referral sources, and used by numerous other interprofessional providers to further understand an individual's performance. This section must be clear, logical, to the point, well supported, complete, and most importantly correct. Given that speech and language evaluations can be quite lengthy and sometimes difficult to understand, the summary section, unfortunately, may be the only part of a report that another busy professional may read. This consideration further underscores the importance of generating a clear and concise summary and impressions section.

A complete speech and language assessment involves hours of face-to-face, or possibly remote, actual testing. Additional hours are added to score, determine result implications, and correlate all of the findings that must be further calculated into the process. There are numerous standardized norm-referenced tests, standardized tests, and criterion-referenced tests, with many of them having subtests that are then used to generate lists and varieties of scores and interpretations. There are authentic assessments, oral peripheral examinations, the case history, and clinical opinions. Many times, a clinician's observation of behavior will become a consideration in the eventual diagnosis. These results must be filtered, condensed, synthesized, and, most importantly, understood by the reader. Strengths and weaknesses of an individual's communication abilities must be determined, and their relative weights and significance must be determined. These results must be seen and explained as they pertain to and support specific areas of communication function. Receptive and expressive language, speech sound production, and pragmatics are a few of the general areas of function that must be considered in any summary and impression presented. Each area assessed in individual tests and their subtests, index scores, results of scales, and informal assessments can provide objective and subjective data to yield information relative to a patient's functioning and eventual diagnosis. Phonological awareness, word retrieval, language organization, attention, memory, and paragraph comprehension are but a fraction of additional areas that potentially may be considered in an assessment. They will be identified as possible areas of strength or weakness. Commonalities, differences, and variations in performance must all be considered as individual pieces of the assessment to be assembled. A picture of the individual being evaluated must be presented considering the reason for the referral, questions being asked, and information presented in the case history. If these pieces are correctly identified and placed together, they will lead to a diagnosis.

WRITING THE SUMMARY

The summary section must provide the reader a review of the pertinent data collected throughout the evaluation and then analyze and synthesize the results in brief, clear, concise statements that "pull" all of the information together. A diagnosis or clinical impression will be supported by the statements provided. The summary should begin with a brief review of the reason the client or patient was referred. If the patient or client was referred with a presenting diagnosis containing relevant medical or academic information, that should also be briefly stated. The summary will then continue highlighting each subsection of the report as to its relevance, important information, and possible relationships to other findings within the report as they lead to a diagnosis or impression.

The summary will then continue with any specific information contained in the case history that will prove relevant to, contribute to, or provide support for the diagnosis or conclusions drawn. Significant findings or information that was revealed in previous reports or stated by an informant might be included as part of the summary.

The determinations of what to include must be made by each evaluator considering their individual importance and contribution toward supporting the conclusions drawn. The importance of each contributing factor must carefully be considered against the length of the summary. The strength and relevance of the information to be included must be weighed. Considerations such as if the case history contains information that is consistent with or conflicts with a diagnosis might be considered as important to include. Similarly, a new diagnosis that is being proposed by the clinician that conflicts with a prior or an existing diagnosis would be an important factor to include in a summary. Reasons would be explained and supported. The skill and experience of the evaluator is once again called on.

A brief description of the client or patient response to testing should be provided to indicate any behavioral aspects that are significant or remarkable and that negatively impacted the performance during the assessment. If the patient was inconsistent in response, distractible, poorly related, or unable to engage in tasks of joint attention, these are examples of behavioral aspects that can be summarized as they can cause barriers to processing information, negatively impact ability to comprehend, impede response, and can be related to a possible diagnosis or needed referral. It is important to differentially diagnose if underlying language ability is being assessed or the deficit lies in an inability to attend. Behavioral concomitants should also be included in a summary if they are associated with specific etiologies to be considered. On the other hand, if the patient was related, cooperative, attentive, and consistent in response, these are relevant markers that should also be noted and very briefly stated.

If an assessment of speech sound production were part of the evaluation, results can be summarized and reported in the summary. There is no need to provide a detailed description of the errors, processes, or substitutions of each of the individual sounds that were problematic or to provide examples in transcribed phrases or sentences. That information is readily available in the body of the report for those who need to see that information. In the summary, it is sufficient to provide the name of a specific test or tests that were administered. Briefly summarize the results and state the nature and severity of any speech sound disorder and additional relevant information as may be noted on the specific test administered. This can be followed by a brief statement indicating the impressions from authentic testing and whether the errors were consistent with the results of standardized assessment. If not, a reason for any discrepancy should be noted with a possible explanation. This is the type of information that is appropriate for the summary and impressions section as it requires analytical thinking based on test results. A diagnosis should be indicated to conclude the brief summary of sound production test results provided. For example, a severe phonological process disorder, childhood apraxia of speech, a mild articulation disorder, or developmentally appropriate speech sound substitutions and distortions should be provided if test results support such diagnoses. If results revealed speech sound production to be within age expectations, as expected for age, or within normal limits, then a simple statement such as "results of formal and informal assessment indicated speech sound production to be age appropriate." A statement regarding overall intelligibility of speech may also be provided such as "overall speech intelligibility during standardized testing and spontaneous speech was age appropriate." In continuing to summarize speech sound production, one should provide a statement regarding stimulability at this point with a statement such as "stimulability for error sounds was good" or "stimulability for error sounds was poor." Information regarding certain aspects of the speech sound assessment is subjective and based on clinical judgments of the evaluator. This is particularly true for overall intelligibility ratings during spontaneous speech and degree of stimulability. The determination of these ratings is clearly done by "impressions" made by the clinician, and that is why they need to be reiterated in the last section of the report as part of the conclusion and tied in with the other overall impressions regarding an individual's communication difficulty.

A statement summarizing the results of an oral peripheral evaluation, if conducted, should be provided based on specific findings and the possible impact on speech sound production or resonance. It is at the evaluator's discretion where the oral peripheral results should be included in the summary and impressions section, in addition to the amount of detail that needs to be provided. This will relate to the specific nature of the initial referral, questions to be answered relative to any structural defect, or functional limitation and diagnosis. In certain evaluations, speech sound production might not be a question and the oral peripheral evaluation may have been done as a routine part of a general examination. If results are unremarkable, it is sufficient to have the information in the body of the report, and a statement regarding the examination would not necessarily warrant space in the summary and impressions. If a clinician, to be thorough, wishes to include this segment of the evaluation, then a simple statement such as "results of an oral peripheral examination were unremarkable," "structure and function of the articulators did not impact on speech sound production," or "oral peripheral articulators were adequate for speech production" makes the point and will suffice.

If relevant anomalies of structure or deficits in function were observed and fully detailed in the body of the report, it is not necessary to again fully describe the findings. Briefly summarize results of the examination and state how they relate to the overall diagnosis. The summary and impressions statement will serve to highlight the finding, explain the significance, and indicate the contribution of the deficit integrated into the summary and impressions of the client or patient's overall functioning. Any support of the findings that adds to establishing a diagnosis or clinical impression should also be provided.

Summarizing the results of language testing is perhaps more complicated for a number of reasons. There are numerous tests involved, each assessing at least one and, more often, many areas of language function. Tests have a variety of scoring mechanisms that are used to explain the results obtained. Composite scores, total test scores, individual subtest scores, core scores, and index scores profiles are examples of the ways test results may be reported psychometrically by test developers. Tests are standardized, standardized norm referenced, and criterion referenced. Many tests for adult disorders such as aphasia or traumatic brain injury compare areas of performance and assess functional ability, and their results can yield profiles that point to specific diagnoses and severities. Authentic testing is also completed where tasks have been described and results presented based on each evaluator's determination. Where does one begin to summarize all of these complex data?

It is helpful to begin by recognizing that all of the complex results, a few of which were previously discussed, are already contained in the body of the report. They should have been presented along with test objectives, types and explanations of scores, and, of course, the actual scores themselves. Examples of errors, results of authentic testing, and charts listing this information should be present. The basic foundation for any language summary has been provided and should be readily accessible in the body of the report. The examiner must now complete the framework that leads to the diagnosis or impression.

The language section of the report, until it is analyzed and synthesized by the clinician, consists of a body of discrete scores that represent the results of numerous decontextualized tasks that were selected to assess numerous areas underlying language function. The tests and tasks selected should have been based on areas that were clinically determined to possibly be indicative of areas of weakness based on interpretation of the reason for referral and case history information. Additional testing was selected by the clinician that was then based on results of the initial tests selected. Those results likely pointed to other discrete areas of language that warranted further exploration. This information, in turn, led to a series of authentic tasks that the evaluator decided would be additionally beneficial in providing information about language that would be gathered in alternative manners. Language function was viewed in nonstandardized, more natural, less decontextualized tasks. There was a logic, process, and connecting thread to the way in which language ability was assessed. The clinician now must view the results of the language assessments to find the connections, common areas of deficit or weakness, and pockets of strengths and weaknesses to best explain why that particular individual was being assessed in the first place. That is what needs to be included in the summary and impressions.

Begin with the standardized test results. The evaluator should analyze the scores from each of the individualized tests administered to determine patterns of consistency. Similarly, these scores should be compared to index scores and other more generalized scores to further assess patterns of strengths and weaknesses. The skilled evaluator will be aware that many omnibus-type assessments and other generalized tests have a great deal of overlap. Receptive and expressive vocabulary, memory, determining multiple meanings of words, following directions, and defining words are but a few of the language areas that are assessed in different ways on many common tests. The evaluator can then analyze patterns of performance across tests and representative tasks. Should patterns of deficit emerge, which usually happens, the task becomes to summarize the representative cores and performance in the functional subareas of language. This should also be done for areas of strength. Scores should be used to indicate levels of severity. The use of standardized test results facilitates this part of the process as it delineates discrete language areas, describes tasks, and provides quantitative data that allow the clinician to readily recognize performance compared to peers or determined criteria.

Once the standardized results have been summarized, the evaluator must then consider the client's or patient's performance on any authentic or dynamic type of assessments utilized. The tasks utilized will have been based on standardized test results, reason for referral, or information contained in the case history. The clinician's analysis of the individual's performance on these assessments will also need to be integrated into the summary. Do the results obtained support the standardized results, indicate better performance than shown in quantitative assessments, or indicate new areas of possible weakness or strength? This integration and synthesis of results is the diagnostic challenge that each evaluator must face. Specifying, explaining, and summarizing this information in written format becomes the additional challenge.

If summarizing the standardized and authentic test results has been carefully and correctly accomplished based on the evaluator's best informed clinical opinion and expertise, the answers to the reason for referral should be apparent. There will be a pattern of weaknesses or deficits and hopefully areas of strengths that should clarify the communication status of the individual being assessed and answer the questions posed in the initial reason for referral. The language summary will provide additional information that will lead to the conclusions and overall impression(s) of the evaluator. The documentation will support any diagnoses or impressions provided. Various deficits and weaknesses in language occur so frequently across the life span that language challenges will be a primary reason for referral for most speech-language pathologists. For toddlers with delayed language to older patients with dementia, and scores of other diagnoses in between, a thorough assessment of language will be required to answer a myriad of referral reasons. The summary of the language assessment as part of an evaluation must be well documented, complete, and well supported. The impressions and conclusions drawn will prove to be a significant section of the speech and language evaluation.

Coding May Be Needed

Coding refers to using a series of defined and recognized "codes" that represent discrete procedures that are directly related to a patient's or client's established diagnoses. An additional, separate set of codes is used to represent the diagnoses related to the procedures performed. The code sets represent the procedures completed and the diagnoses under which they are performed as provided by medical and allied health providers. Codes are largely used by insurance companies and other relevant stakeholders and researchers to input, organize, compare, manage, manipulate, and store medical information in computer systems for a variety of reasons. Using a series of letters and numbers, the diagnosis or problem addressed and "what was done" for them can be inputted into a patient's or client's records and filtered out in a universally understood manner. The coding system also provides for "modifiers" to be added to the codes that further indicate information including the manner in which therapy was provided (e.g., remote) or units of time spent. This system is a critical foundation of medical recordkeeping and is essential to reimbursement for services provided. It is increasingly more important with electronic health recordkeeping and the rapidly occurring data shift from paper to computer that is well under way.

Coding for Speech-Language Pathology

Speech and language evaluators may be asked to add "codes" to their evaluations, which may usually be added in the summary and impressions section. If not included in the actual report, it will certainly be needed for insurance reimbursement purposes.

Medicaid, Medicare, and third-party payers require this for reimbursement and are very strict in monitoring, verifying, and even auditing these codes and reimbursements. Early Intervention and certain therapies provided through school systems can be reimbursed for services through various entities and often require codes. Speech-language pathologists must be knowledgeable in this area as not providing codes or using incorrect codes will result in denial of reimbursement or approval for service.

The coding for the procedures performed by clinicians, as well as other medical providers, is most frequently specified under the Current Procedural Terminology (CPT) system. There are codes to specify the evaluation processes and, more specifically, CPT codes for what was actually evaluated such as speech or fluency. CPT codes are also used to indicate individual or group therapy sessions. Modifiers are also used such as utilizing "-95" following a CPT code to indicate the session was provided remotely via teletherapy. A second system, the International Classification of Diseases-10-CM (ICD-10), is used to specify the disorder that is being evaluated or treated. The 10th edition is currently used (American Medical Association, 2016; American Speech-Language-Hearing Association, n.d.b).

According to the Centers for Disease Control and Prevention, the United States developed a Clinical Modification (ICD-10-CM) for medical diagnoses based on the World Health Organization's (WHO) ICD-10, and the Centers for Medicare & Medicaid Services developed a new Procedure Coding System (ICD-10-PCS) for inpatient procedures. There are thousands of diagnostic codes that are revised as new editions are made available. These diagnostic codes are used for a variety of reasons, including maintaining health statistics, research, measuring outcomes, tracking public health, billing, and claims reimbursement.

The *Diagnostic and Statistical Manual of Mental Disorders, Fifth Edition* (DSM-5) is also used for coding diagnoses. According to the American Psychiatric Association (2013), "The *Diagnostic and Statistical Manual of Mental Disorders* is the handbook used by health care professionals in the United States and much of the world as the authoritative guide to the diagnosis of mental disorders." The DSM-5 contains descriptions, symptoms, and other criteria for diagnosing mental disorders. It provides a common language for clinicians to communicate about their patients and establishes consistent and reliable diagnoses that can be used in the research of mental disorders (APA, n.d.). The DSM-5 coding system is in use by insurance companies and may be viewed as a companion to the ICD-10.

This summary is provided to inform readers of another aspect of diagnostic report writing of which they need to be aware. ASHA (n.d.-a) provides helpful detailed coding information for clinicians on its website. There are continuing education courses, books, and other resources that cover this topic. An example of coding information for a speech and language evaluation (ASHA, n.d.c) to assess a child's language may be presented in a report as follows:

- CPT-92523: Evaluation of Speech Sound Production With Evaluation of Language and Comprehension
- ICD-10-CM: F80.2 Mixed Receptive-Expressive Language Disorder

If the evaluation was provided remotely via telepractice and the diagnosis was aphasia, the accepted codes would look like this:

- CPT-96105-95: Evaluation of Aphasia (Language)
- ICD-10-CM: I69.320 Aphasia

While these two code sets appear simple and straightforward, the skill and knowledge to provide them should not be underestimated. The information to support the diagnosis must be provided in the diagnostic evaluation, and the evaluator must be prepared to support their determination if questioned.

Lastly, the reader should be aware that ASHA recognizes the WHO International Classification of Functioning, Disability and Health (Blake & McLeod, 2018) as a coding system that can be applied to speech, language, and hearing disorders. There are numerous references on ASHA's website, and other resources are available for clinicians who desire to learn more about this system. Specific accountable and knowledgeable coding is an essential part of the diagnostic process, reporting, and documentation for any clinician.

REFERENCES

American Medical Association. (2016). *About CPT coding.* https://www.ama-assn.org/practice-management/cpt-current-procedural-terminology/

American Psychiatric Association. (n.d.). *DSM-5: Frequently asked questions.* https://www.psychiatry.org

American Psychiatric Association. (2013). *Diagnostic and statistical manual of mental disorders* (5th ed.).

American Speech-Language-Hearing Association. (n.d.-a). *About ICD-10-CM coding for audiology and speech pathology.* https://www.asha.org/practice/reimbursement/coding/

American Speech-Language-Hearing Association. (n.d.-b). *Coding for reimbursement.* https://www.asha.org/practice/reimbursement/coding/

American Speech-Language-Hearing Association. (n.d.-c). *Current procedural terminology (CPT) codes.* https://www.asha.org/practice/reimbursement/coding/

Blake, H., & McLeod, S. (2018). *The International Classification of Functioning, Disability and Health: Considering individuals from a perspective of health and wellness: Perspectives of the ASHA special interest groups.* https://doi.org/10.1044/persp3.SIG17.69

Centers for Disease Control and Prevention. (n.d.). https://www.cdc.gov

Recommendations and Referrals
What It's All About, so Write It Right

You're almost finished! You've considered the reasons for the referral and the case history information. The testing has been completed and scored, and the results have been analyzed. You've integrated and summarized the results to support a diagnosis and impression. Most of the work to complete the evaluation has been done, and now it is time to complete the last part of the report. It continues to require the same analytical thinking, skills, and knowledge that were used throughout the diagnostic process. This is the last critical element in the diagnostic report writing process, and the decisions made here must be clear, clinically supported in the report, and well expressed. The only thing that remains will be your signature. The clinician must now provide recommendations for any suggested therapies or interventions and provide all of the necessary interprofessional referrals to other specialists. Additional evaluations for other possible interventions by those other than speech-language pathologists may be called for, explained, and rationales provided. The clinician may also provide considerations for specific school settings, placements, or sites that could provide the appropriate therapeutic resources and support as needed by the client or patient assessed. These recommendations and referrals provide the experienced clinician the opportunity to demonstrate their expertise in yet another area of the evaluation process. This all must be carefully documented. The skill set involved in determining recommendations and referrals relies on intuition, experience, and a deep understanding of available resources, therapeutic possibilities, specialized interventions,

Blaustein, S. H. *Diagnostic Report Writing in Speech–Language Pathology: A Guide to Effective Communication* (pp. 107–115). © 2023 Taylor & Francis Group.

and assessments across disciplines. These referrals and recommendations must also often consider rules, regulations, qualifying characteristics, and possible reimbursement sources.

The recommendations and referrals made must be individualized and based on each client's or patient's reason for the referral, case history, assessment results, and diagnosis. This section cannot rely on a template, rote, or "boilerplate" formula for a universal set of recommendations and referrals that is always "typically" used. The precise recommendations and referrals will vary as widely as each individual being assessed.

Recommendations for Making Recommendations

Just as the reason for the referral and case history information drives the plan for the evaluation, the summary, diagnosis, and diagnostic impression(s) drive the determination for the necessary recommendations and referrals to be made.

First, the evaluator must determine whether there is a need to provide speech or language therapy for any communication disorder that may have been diagnosed. This decision should fall within the clinician's area of competence if they are completing speech and language assessments. If the evaluator decides that therapy is to be recommended, that must clearly be stated. There are then a number of additional factors that follow and must be specified. The determination of the need for therapy will be a decision made based on the experience and expertise of the evaluator after considering the evaluation in its entirety. There are few, if any, objective indices that draw a clear line between recommending or not recommending therapy. For a moderate or severe communication disorder, this determination is often very clear and easy to make. For other cases, the decision to recommend therapy may not be as straightforward. Less severe cases, whether a problem may resolve with time, impact on the individual, considerations of a child's developmental level and chronological age, or whether or not to be proactive are but a few of the variables that can make recommending therapy more difficult. It is here that principles of evidence-based practice such as clinician's judgment or wishes of a patient, client, or family come into play. These sources are often more relied on than determinations based on randomly controlled trials and research, the highest levels of evidence-based practice. Once the need for therapy has been clearly decided by the clinician, the following additional factors can then be taken into careful consideration, detailed, and documented.

1. **Frequency.** Frequency refers to the number of sessions of intervention over a time period. The clinician must determine and specify and recommend how often a client or patient should be seen. Should this be once per week, twice per week, or, for some reason, biweekly? This number must be provided and is at the discretion of the evaluating clinician.

2. **Duration.** How long should each therapy session be? The evaluator must provide the recommended time length of each session. The most common durations are 30, 45, or 60 minutes per session. Considerations will include the tolerance level of the client or patient, frustration levels, age, attention span, availability of services, and service delivery models of those providing the services. While a clinician may recommend a specific duration, the final decision may ultimately be out of the evaluator's hands. This includes frequency as well. Whatever extrinsic factors may be involved, a recommendation for duration must be made. There is emerging literature beginning to discuss frequencies and durations of therapy for various disorders in consideration of many factors, including principles of motor learning and practice. Any clinician providing evaluations should be familiar with this emerging literature.

3. **Group size.** The clinician must specify if the patient or client should be seen individually or in a group. There are reasons to recommend both types of settings. Individualized therapy may be more suitable and have advantages for certain types of therapies and disorders where more specific and individually tailored interventions are necessary. Group therapy is usually recommended where there is a need for developing social skills, discourse, targeted peer interventions, or play. Considerations for placing adults in group settings may include the above but also have more dynamic reasons such

as providing peer support and opportunities to create relationships with individuals and their families in similar situations. Group therapy may also be recommended for scheduling reasons where individuals with similar disorders and/or goals can be seen in homogeneous or heterogeneous groups for a variety of reasons. Considerations frankly may take into account staff availability, budget, or space. These are not the best reasons to recommend group vs. individual therapy, and if challenged, it may be hard to justify these reasons clinically. When groups are recommended, it should be realized that individual dosage can be reduced. Dosage refers to the actual one-on-one time of actual intervention that a client or patient is receiving. When a group is recommended, the number of individuals in the group should be clearly specified. The recommendation may include a dyad or a specific number such as 3 or 4. A maximum group size may also be provided. Rationales for these decisions should be stated if possible.

4. **Specific therapeutic interventions.** There are times based on the disorder diagnosed, impression, or results of the evaluation that a specific technique or approach would be the preferred method for a particular client or individual. This will be based on the knowledge, experience, and intuition of the clinician completing the evaluation. These specific recommendations might involve a general technique or strategy but also involve a recognized, often evidence-based intervention for a specific communication disorder. The ability to make this type of recommendation is within the scope of practice of the speech-language pathologist completing the assessment. Common approaches, interventions, or techniques may include Prompts for Reorganizing Oral Motor Targets (PROMPT), the Silverman Voice Method for patients with Parkinson's disease, the Picture Exchange Communication System (PECS), or other specific augmentative and alternative communication (AAC) approaches. Consideration of a variety of techniques for voice therapies or approaches to fluency is another area that would be within the scope of practice for the assessing speech-language pathologist to provide a specific recommendation. The clinician should also be aware that under some conditions, such as evaluations within a school district, the speech-language pathologist may not be permitted to recommend a specific approach or therapy technique. It should also be realized that while a clinician is free to make these recommendations, they may not necessarily be followed by a treating clinician, readily available, or funded by a third-party payer. Recommendations, however appropriate and correct, are just that: recommendations. This should not deter an evaluator, if permitted, to provide all of the necessary recommendations for interventions as part of their report. The clinician, after all, has done the assessment, should understand the patient or client, and have a clear idea of what approach may work best for an individual considering all facets of the assessment.

5. **Speech or language therapy not recommended.** Speech or language therapy may not always be recommended. The results of the evaluation may indicate that the client or patient's communication skills may be at or close to age expectations. The original reason for the referral may have raised a question or concern that turns out to be less serious than in reality, developmentally appropriate as it presents, or within another professional's scope of practice. The evaluator may for a variety of reasons not recommend speech or language intervention. The report will indicate that after thorough consideration of the results of the assessment, the communication levels of the individual being evaluated are "within expectations" or "There are no clinically significant communication deficits, weaknesses, or difficulties." The clinician should be comfortable in stating "speech and/or language therapy is not recommended at this time." Similarly, if there is a reason to believe that because of a younger individual's age, continued concerns of the patient or client, or a desire to monitor the patient over time, it may also be appropriate to recommend a reevaluation within a specified time interval. In that case, a statement such as "a re-evaluation in 6 months is recommended." It would also be appropriate and advisable in such a case that the evaluator remains available to the client, patient, or family. This should also be documented in a statement such as "should additional concerns be noted or any further questions arise regarding communication skills, it is recommended that the evaluator be contacted before 6 months or as needed."

6. **Delay initiation of speech or language therapy.** There are cases where therapy is recommended, but for some reason, it is suggested by the evaluator that the initiation of therapy be delayed. This may be as simple as a child in need of articulation therapy but developmentally may be missing necessary dentition that would better facilitate teaching the sounds in question. A recommendation to wait until dental structure matures or develops could be appropriate. Waiting to commence therapy could also apply to other structural anomalies that have occurred in both adults and children for a variety of reasons. Intervention may be recommended, but further completion of surgical procedures, provision of prosthetics, consideration of orthodontia, or other medical reasons may preclude starting immediately or soon after the evaluation. This should be documented with the evaluator's recommendation for therapy clearly indicated with an additional recommendation to delay therapy initiation for the specific rationale explained.

Speech or language therapy could be indicated for a client or patient who may not have the prerequisite behavioral set to attend to tasks, comply, or participate in the therapeutic process. It can be very frustrating for both the client or patient and the treating therapist to provide therapy in such cases. Therapy, although needed, might in fact be contraindicated for a variety of behavioral reasons. A recommendation for speech therapy or language therapy if needed is appropriate and should be documented, but recommendations might also include that "interfering behavioral concomitant should be first evaluated and possibly addressed." This would ultimately make the speech and language intervention more successful. Consideration of evidence-based practice fundamentals indicates that family concerns and considerations also be taken into account in our assessment and intervention processes. If a family indicates they are unable to practice with an individual at home, reliably get the individual to therapy sessions, or implement recommendations for environmental modifications, these types of reasons should be considered and addressed in the recommendation. These types of considerations might necessitate delaying, modifying, or adjusting frequency of therapy and may be advisable and justifiable.

7. **Recommend counseling.** Speech-language pathologists should remember that counseling is within their scope of practice. It is an important aspect of our interventions and can be a critical adjunct to the therapies we provide. There are numerous books, continuing education programs, graduate-level courses, journal articles, workshops, and online courses that deal with the aspect of counseling patients or clients with communication disorders. Family members, caregivers, friends, or partners can also be involved in the counseling process. If the evaluator feels for any reason that counseling is an appropriate recommendation, it should be specifically mentioned and documented as a recommendation. The type of counseling, specific areas, topics or subjects to be discussed, and who should be counseled should be in the recommendation. A recommendation, if needed, may even specify the type of counselor. If there is a need for adaptations, environmental modifications, modifying communication of those around the client or patient, or use of visual or other supports, this should also be discussed. These types of recommendations may be provided through counseling to the individuals surrounding the client or patient. The client or patient themselves may need to be counseled regarding the nature, extent, and implications of their communication disorder, and behavioral and emotional reaction should be considered. If counseling of a more in-depth dynamic is needed or as the result of more significant factors such as depression or anxiety, a recommendation should be made through an appropriate referral.

The previous discussion provides an introduction into the need for consultation with, assessment by, or intervention from professionals from other disciplines. This highlights the need for interprofessional practice (IPP) that has been discussed previously. Cotreating an individual in need of speech or language therapy with the assistance of other appropriate professionals who can provide behavioral, emotional, pharmacological, medical, and other support is not unusual. It speaks to the importance of and need for recognizing IPP.

In summary, recommendations for speech, language, voice, fluency, or other related services provided by speech-language pathologists within their scope of practice must be given careful consideration. Providing, approving, accepting, and funding therapy, if necessary, is the next step that

TABLE 12-1
Factors to Be Addressed in Recommending Interventions
• Individual vs. group therapy
• Group size: specific number or maximum group size
• Duration of therapy sessions
• Frequency of therapy sessions
• Location of therapy services: push-in vs. pull-out; office/home
• Rationales for interventions recommended
• Special qualifications/certifications of providers
• Specific types of interventions/techniques

follows the evaluation process. The clearer and more specific the recommendations are written and provided in the diagnostic evaluation, the easier it will be to successfully clear the hurdles. Table 12-1 lists many of the basic components that must be decided on and documented. There is some but not a large body of evidence-based data to support many of these choices. The evaluator must analyze the evaluation results, provide the best recommendations based on available data, document them, and stand behind them!

MAKING REFERRALS: INTERPROFESSIONAL PRACTICE IS GOOD PRACTICE

IPP has never been more important in the practice of speech-language pathology. While the term "interprofessional" in and of itself suggests what it may involve, a clear and thorough understanding of the core components and principles of IPP is essential to a speech-language pathologist who is providing assessment and intervention for individuals with communication disorders. While any clinician would say that they are familiar with multidisciplinary practice and have even participated as part of a "team," the current understanding of recognized IPP principles must be realized as a concept apart, and more theoretically complex, than a few different specialists treating the same client or patient. The reader is directed to the website of the American Speech-Language-Hearing Association (ASHA) as a resource to fully understand IPP as it is currently understood. Principles, concepts, and core ideas are put into perspective, and additional resources and references are provided. There are currently numerous additional opportunities and available resources to learn about IPP.

"Scope of practice" is the term that indicates what we as speech-language pathologists are trained to do, licensed to do, and capable and competent in doing. The ASHA Code of Ethics states that we must always practice within our "scope of practice." The reasons for this will not be discussed here but should be obvious. Suffice it to say that there are other disciplines where other professionals are specifically trained, certified, credentialed, licensed, and experienced to better provide interprofessional evaluations and interventions than we are. There are limits to what we may clinically provide under our scope of practice. This concept also applies to certain assessments and interventions that we are technically capable of doing and exist within our scope of practice, but an evaluator may not have the experience, training, or competency to perform. Recognizing this important consideration is one factor that leads to providing appropriate referrals as part of our diagnostic report writing process. The referral process can also be seen as another logical construct that can be understood across assessments. The following should be considered when determining what referrals to recommend.

1. **Decide what information may be missing from the assessment.** Is there anything else that you need to know that, for any reason, you are unable to determine? Does another professional need to do a further assessment to provide the "missing pieces?" It is necessary to determine any missing aspects of the evaluation that are needed to fully answer the questions raised in the reason for referral, confirm a possible diagnosis, or rule out a confounding diagnosis? There may be questions about an individual's communication process that can be impacted by medical reasons, structure, attentional reasons, neurological reasons, or any other possible contributing factors that are beyond our scope of practice to evaluate. If that is the case, a referral must be made to the appropriate professional for assessment of the specific area in question. The reason for the referral should be clearly explained.

2. **Decide if any specific techniques or interventions may be needed for the client or patient by other professionals.** As part of the recommendation process, an intervention may be deemed necessary and a referral must be made to another professional who may be better suited to decide on the appropriateness of that intervention for your client or patient. As part of the interdisciplinary process, it is not unusual for a speech-language pathologist to "cotreat" with other professionals providing interventions in different specialty areas that will facilitate overall improvement of function for an individual. This is subtly different from the previous discussion as the referral is specifically with respect to whether a recommended intervention would be helpful for the particular individual being assessed. This referral may actually be to another speech-language pathologist with a specialty in areas such as feeding, PROMPT, AAC, or other interventions where specialized training or certification is required. The evaluating clinician may have sufficient expertise to know that a certain client or patient may benefit from a certain approach but needs confirmation from a provider with the proper credentials, training, and experience to make the final determination. There should be no reason for concern to admit that there are other professionals within our own profession who should be sought for additional information. The referral would include that the reason for the referral is to confirm whether in the opinion of the other professional the recommended therapy or intervention would be appropriate and beneficial for the individual in question. Similar referrals are made for applied behavioral analysis (ABA) sensory interventions, occupational therapy, academic areas in the case of dyslexia, or other relevant associated therapies where an interdisciplinary approach toward intervention would be beneficial.

3. **Decide on the type of interprofessional referral that best meets the needs of the client or patient.** Many disciplines overlap. If a patient needs to be seen to rule out a possible diagnosis of autism spectrum disorder, a referral may be made to any number of professionals. A neuropsychologist, developmental pediatrician, psychiatrist, child psychologist, or pediatric neurologist all may be capable of doing the necessary assessment. In certain cases, a referral may be made to more than one professional to confirm a diagnosis. The evaluating clinician is reminded that it can suffice to specify the type of referral that is needed, information sought, and rationale for seeking that information. The name of a specific professional does not need to be and should not be placed in the report. There is an additional consideration in actually making referrals to specific other individuals by name that is different from recommending the type of the evaluation that is required. Suffice it to say that the evaluator, if asked to make a specific referral, which often happens, should be aware of ethical, professional, and legal ramifications. There are numerous professional issues that can arise from providing inappropriate referral sources. Table 12-2 lists examples of professionals across disciplines that speech-language pathologists, depending on employment setting, refer to interprofessionally. The list is quite extensive, and there can be others depending on specialized needs.

4. **Be sure to provide, clarify, and explain the specific type of referral recommended.** When making a referral, the specific information being sought, reason for the referral, and any supporting information the referring evaluator can provide will be helpful to the person receiving the referral. It is often beneficial if the referral source will actually have a copy of the evaluator's report or at least a summary letter explaining the referral. This documents the referral and avoids any misunderstanding or incorrect reasons provided by the client, caregivers, or family to explain the reason for the

TABLE 12-2
Examples of Interprofessional Referrals Made by Speech-Language Pathologists

• Audiologist	• Otolaryngologist
• Board-certified behavior analyst	• Pediatric neurologist
• Developmental pediatrician	• Physical therapist
• Educational/reading specialist	• Plastic surgeon
• Geneticist	• Prosthodontist
• Neurologist	• Psychiatrist
• Neuropsychologist	• Psychologist
• Occupational therapist	• Psychopharmacologist
• Oral surgeon	• Social worker
• Orthodontist	• Technology support/AAC specialist

referral. The author has often had individuals referred for speech or language evaluations as part of another interdisciplinary evaluation where the reason for the referral was unclear. It was difficult to determine from the patient, client, or informants specifically the information that was being sought. Being clear in documenting the referrals eliminates confusion, incorrect assessments, and unnecessary assessments and avoids the clinician having to directly contact the referral source. Just as scope of practice of professionals can overlap, the type of assessments and actual tests done may overlap. It is not unusual for a neuropsychologist to use many of the language tests that are also used by speech-language pathologists. Speech-language pathologists may use tests that are common to psychologists, neuropsychologists, or reading specialists. Clarity in referral can avoid duplicating administration of tests. The author has observed this occurring, and clarity in referrals and providing as much information as possible along with the referral can eliminate this problem.

A Very Important Finale

As with every other part of the evaluation, the recommendations and referrals section is extremely important, carries weight, and should be correct and well documented. Following completion of a thorough, well-documented evaluation of communication functioning, determining the appropriate recommendations and referrals based on correct diagnostic impressions is critical. The client or patient will value the suggestions provided, follow up on them, or perhaps seek second opinions or consultations prior to implementing them. Determining and providing these important steps in the diagnostic process is what the client or individual came for in the first place. The recommendations should be carefully thought out, based on information determined during the assessment and in consideration of the reason for referral and case history. They must follow careful analysis and thought. Referrals are made for specific reasons, to complete unfinished aspects of the evaluation process, to obtain additional needed information, and to consider other therapies or interventions and any other number of reasons. These recommendations and referrals will often take time to put into place, as well as involve travel and expense. They can often produce anxiety as one moves through the process and awaits results. This final section should be clear, well thought out, supported, and specific.

Recommendations will be viewed and considered by numerous individuals beyond the client or patient. These are the parties that make critical decisions involving provision of services, qualifications for placements, determination of classroom setting, adult rehabilitation settings, and other critical decisions. Individuals reading the recommendations will be in positions to approve funding. Recommendations should be logical, convincing, necessary, and based on clinical evidence. As previously discussed, the clinician should be aware of the necessary determinants to have the recommendations approved where necessary. The required information to obtain approvals must be present.

Referrals are viewed by others in our own professional community and interprofessionally. Seeking outside assessment for additional information or considerations for interventions speaks to our judgment and competency as evaluators. It reflects on who we are as professionals. As in other parts of the entire diagnostic and report writing process, the steps detailed in this section are not unique to a specific diagnosis. Understanding the general concepts involved in this part of the process will generalize to other diagnoses.

Whether evaluating an individual with aphasia, a child with a possible learning disability or attention-deficit disorder, or an adolescent who stutters, recommendations and referrals will need to be made. The general considerations and processes for determining recommendations and referrals cross diagnostic lines. What changes is the specificity related to each diagnosis. This concept should be useful to diagnostic report writers.

The bulk of the clinical work involved in the diagnostic process and subsequent documentation has led to this point. This is not the section of the report, as with all sections, to take less time, less thought, or less analysis. It is not the "easy part." It is far better that you have clients or patients provide feedback thanking the clinician for correct recommendations and referrals than to have feedback where the therapist may have missed a necessary referral or made an inappropriate recommendation. This author has received emails, calls, texts, and letters where a parent or the individual themself has expressed gratitude for the right recommendation or referral that has made a huge difference in an individual's life. This occurs following significant graduations, employments, and achievements that were never thought possible at the time of the evaluation. This is the type of feedback that is incredibly rewarding and speaks to the challenges and excitement that can be just one part of the diagnostic and documentation process.

NOTES ON SIGNATURES

As stated previously in this book, each report will bear the clinician's signature at the conclusion. It certifies that the name that appears is the person responsible for the content of the report from start to finish. Little is written about how to sign a report, and again, there is no standard way specified. Various work settings, for uniformity, may specify how a report is to be signed and what information should be included. Thus, varied formats exist. The standard way to sign a document would be to type the individual's name and title with a signature above the printed name. Credentials are often used. Thus, a signature might appear as:

Mary Smith, PhD, CCC-SP, BCS-CL
Speech-Language Pathologist

This indicates that Mary Smith holds a doctorate degree, has a Certificate of Clinical Competence in Speech Pathology, and is a Board-Certified Specialist in Child Language. Dr. Smith's job title is speech-language pathologist. In some instances a state license and number may be required. This signature is professional, is well presented, and contains basic essential information.

Numerous variations are seen from report to report. In some cases, the credentials indicated by the abbreviations are spelled out under the signature. As most individuals may not be familiar with the credentialing used by ASHA and other institutions or agencies, the explanation can prove helpful. More specific titles such as chairperson, supervisor, chief, or senior can be added if appropriate.

If a student contributed to an evaluation, their signature should appear indicating they are a student clinician. The report is then cosigned by the supervising, certified speech-language pathologist. This may also hold true for clinicians during their Clinical Fellowship. Signatures have legal status, and their use should be carefully monitored to be correctly included.

There are a few caveats to be aware of with respect to formatting and providing signatures. This author has seen numerous signatures throughout the years where clinicians have added their own titles. Examples include "Articulation Specialist, Specializing in Stuttering or Specialist in Voice Disorders." While this may be true, one has to be careful not to infer that there is a type of credential, certificate, or degree that is held. This can be confusing as ASHA increases the use of "specialty recognition" programs. Similarly, clinicians often include committees served on, offices held, or other similar accomplishments. One has to consider the function of the signature, their title, and role in signing the document. One also has to carefully question the need to add additional layers to "pad" a title if the roles are not necessarily directly related to the report or will in some manner add value to the report for eventual readers. It is a report, not a résumé.

Clinicians should also be aware of "cross-titling." If one were to complete an evaluation under the auspices and their role at a university clinic, even as a supervisor, it makes sense to include a title such as "Associate Professor" indicating the department and name of the university. If, however, the same clinician completes a private evaluation in a private office, without any connection to the university or their role there, other questions are raised. By including the name and title of an additional setting in a private report, to what degree would the university be involved should there be a complaint, suit, or action? Again, reports have legal status, and these issues should be carefully explored and clarified by appropriate professionals if there is any question.

Last, with constant updates in technology, traditional tasks such as simple signatures on reports and documents must be reexamined. Use of computers, electronic health recordkeeping, and instant transfer of information has necessitated numerous changes in tasks as previously as simple as signing a report. Clinicians are advised to keep abreast of this ever-changing technology, including sending reports with the clinician's signature transmitted electronically or the use of having clients or patients signing important forms remotely. Numerous programs are now readily available that allow an individual to sign a document "online," and there is an ever-increasing use of this technology. Rules and regulations may vary by state, and clinicians are advised to realize the benefits and risks that may be involved in using this technology in their practice. In recognizing gender diversity individuals across settings have recently added identifying pronouns to their signature field. This is a matter of choice and one should be aware of work setting policy in this area.

One More Read

10 Common Errors in Report Writing to Avoid

As careful as an evaluator can be in preparing a diagnostic report and with as many reports as one has completed, reports still are uploaded, mailed, or distributed with mistakes. These can vary from one error to a few and an insignificant minor error where a word is deleted to more significant errors in scoring, including incorrect information, or deleting critical data. Suffice it to say that it should not happen but it does for a variety of reasons. These range from carelessness to distraction to technical errors in preparation or transmission. When errors occur in a diagnostic, all one can do is deal with it on a case-by-case basis, honestly, ethically, and quickly to reduce any negative outcomes as a result. Specific recommendations cannot be provided as to the unpredictability of when and why they occur. A last careful read of each evaluation is always warranted with the following final points kept in mind.

1. Errors of Spelling and Grammar

Too often reports may be completed and sent to referral sources, parents, agencies, or requesting bodies that contain errors of spelling, grammar, punctuation, or awkward language. This is easy to avoid by taking the time to proofread and spell checking to make sure that each report reflects the highest professional standards and yourself as an evaluator.

Blaustein, S. H. *Diagnostic Report Writing in Speech–Language Pathology: A Guide to Effective Communication* (pp. 117-120).

2. Overuse and Reliance on Templates

It is very easy given the redundancy that is involved in certain aspects of report writing to rely on templates to save time and facilitate the report writing process. This is especially true of computer-generated reports that are now widely available with online scoring available, including written results, test details, and summaries. Admittedly, there are segments of reports that may allow a basic skeleton template where scores or other core information can be input. If used, extreme care must be taken to ensure that the information is correct and the report is completely individualized. This includes every aspect of the report with special care given to individualized summary, impressions, results, recommendations, and referrals. The author has been involved in meetings, hearings, and appeals where templates have obviously been used by the evaluator. This is easily determined when a wrong name appears in a report, genders are confused, languages spoken or dates of birth and ages are incorrect. The author has also heard administrators from school districts state during meetings "these are the same recommendations this evaluator provides in every report we have seen." It is difficult to respect the integrity and validity of a report where it is obvious a template has been used and a report was completed by just "filling in the blanks." This is unprofessional and the ethics must be questioned at times.

3. Having Incorrect Information in the Case History

Case histories can often be detailed and complex. They are content heavy with dates, sequences, events, and sometimes the names of disorders or pathologies, many of which can be uncommon. An evaluator should check with informants and documents provided if there is any question as to the integrity and correctness of any information contained. It is easier to avoid errors such as these before reports are completed and distributed than to have it pointed out by referral sources or clients or patients who call or email to correct information that was contained in a completed report. Again, if one part of a report is questionable, it can lead to an inference that other parts of the report may be questionable as well.

4. Omission of Required Content for the Purpose of the Report

As discussed in this book, various reports are not only written to evaluate a patient but also contain the necessary information and recommendations that are needed for the myriad purposes our evaluations and reports serve. The evaluator should always keep in mind the numerous reasons that reports are written beyond basic assessment and diagnosis of a client or patient. It is time-consuming to receive feedback from a client, insurance company, or any one of a number of types of representatives that approve placements and services that needed information that was not contained in the report. This is especially frustrating when the information was available as a result of the evaluation but for some reason not included in the report. Be certain completed reports contain all of the necessary information at every level.

5. Forgetting the "Small Stuff"

In addition to completing our reports, there is often necessary accompanying paperwork that is required. This includes Health Insurance Portability and Accountability Act forms, insurance forms, releases, addresses, and biographical data forms. Forgetting these forms, neglecting them, and not making sure they are complete and signed leads to having to contact clients or patients or their families or guardians to obtain the necessary documents before a report goes out. Contacting patients after evaluations have been completed for this type of documentation can again be indicative of a lack of detail or error. It is far better to have all of the paperwork completed as required.

6. Not Doing the Math

Errors in adding raw scores or total test scores, not correctly using all subtests in index scores, not determining correct chronological age when the birth date is correct, and not recognizing or incorrectly using basals and ceilings during testing are but a few of the errors that can lead to gross errors in final test results. A small error in addition in determining a raw score can result in a significant error in a final percentile or standard deviation attained. Incorrect addition of scale scores to find an index score or elimination or addition of one of the necessary subtest scores contained in a total test score or index score can also result in significant errors in test results. This author has been involved in circumstances where all of these types of errors have occurred and been pointed out at hearings or meetings. Again, this not only reflects on the competence of the evaluator but adversely impacts results and needs of the client or patient. Once the accuracy incompetency of the evaluator is brought to question, the recommendations and referrals can also be easily questioned.

7. Forgetting the Importance of Timelines and Dates

Reports may have timelines and deadlines associated with them. Evaluations by school districts to determine Individualized Education Plans and insurance companies often indicate that the case will be closed unless a response or an evaluation is received by a specific date. It is important that an evaluator is aware whenever a report is needed by a certain date. The clinician should be certain they can complete the assessment, as well as have the report written, including sending it to the requested recipient, within the timeline requested by the patient, client, or representative. If an evaluator cannot complete the evaluation within the time frame requested, they should decline the evaluation. Rushing through an evaluation, not completing all tests, or reducing testing to save time and rushing through scoring and analysis can only result in errors. Working hours to complete a report along with other responsibilities to have the report ready by the deadline can be overwhelming and stressful and should be avoided. Missing deadlines, last-minute hurried reports, or getting repeated phone calls questioning "where is the report" can be avoided with proper time management and organization. It is fair and considerate to all of those involved in the assessment process to indicate before accepting an evaluation if it cannot be completed appropriately within the requested time interval.

8. Forgetting to Ask Yourself the Important Questions

Remembering the basic questions that one should be asking themselves throughout the report writing process is important. In getting involved in the details involved in assessing, diagnosing, and report writing, it can be easy to forget the essential elements. Always ask, "Is this correct, relevant, defensible, important, and accurate?"

Is this stated in the correct and most efficient language? Is it complete and error free? Answering yes to all of these questions will result in better report writing.

9. Lack of Clarity and Specificity in Recommendations

The recommendation specified by the evaluator must be considered by the eventual end users of the report. If they are not clear, specific, and reasonable, they will be difficult to have approved. When recommending interventions, there are numerous considerations. Is the frequency of therapy specified? Is the duration of each session clear? Is it individual or group? How many in a group? Who is to provide the therapy? Should the therapist have any special certifications or qualifications? Is there a specific type of intervention that is recommended? This all needs to be supported in the summary and impressions. "Starting speech therapy is recommended" or "language therapy is recommended weekly" is not a sufficient recommendation.

In some cases, it can even be asked if the evaluator is the one to make the recommendations. Not all settings allow the evaluator to make specific recommendations or referrals. They may need to be determined during another meeting or planning session or require interprofessional consensus.

10. Not Considering and Making Appropriate Referrals

In the current clinical environment where interprofessional practice is becoming paramount across disciplines in providing the best patient and client care, it is essential to determine if additional evaluations, assessments, and interventions will be needed. Many speech, language, and swallowing disorders are associated with broader conditions, diseases, and pathologies that are not limited solely to communication. Disorders of communication, including subtle changes in voice, sound production, or word finding, can be early indicators of more severe systemic underlying conditions that must be confirmed, ruled out, or in need of other interventions. Failure to make appropriate referral recommendations is not in the best interest of the patient, can lead to delayed diagnosis, and, in extreme cases, can be considered a form of malpractice.

INDEX